STEWART NORDENSSON
1937-1999

Stewart Nordensson, co-author of the Teamwork books
died on October 5, 1999. This printing and all
future printings of Teamwork are lovingly
dedicated to his memory.

ACKNOWLEDGEMENTS

The authors wish to thank many people for their help in making this project succeed.

Very special thanks go to Jeff Nordensson for giving me the computers and equipment that not only made it possible for me to dictate my thoughts but also opened up a whole new way of communicating all over the world.

Many years ago, I was having trouble with a nine-week old Belgian tervuren puppy. Donna, my late wife, asked, "Who is the Top Dog anyway?" I said, "Thank you, Honey, I have been trying to think of a name for this new organization." Without TOP DOG, you wouldn't be reading this book. It's the place where we put our ideas into practice and that's why we know they work. It's the staff that spent many hours researching and finding the money and the printer to make this book real. It's many colleagues who read the early manuscripts and offered invaluable suggestions. Thank you, TOP DOG.

Thank you to everyone who showed up at different times and places to have your pictures taken, and thank you for allowing us to publish your names and photographs so that everyone can see how you succeeded.

Special thanks to Scott Ash, our photographer, who donated much time and energy to this project.

Thanks to all the people at Nordensson Lynn & Associates, Inc. who generously gave of their time to turn the manuscript into a real book, with special thanks to Jeff, David, Denice, Renee and Maureen.

And thanks to the thousands of people with disabilities who would like to have a well behaved dog and believe they have the ability to make it happen. If we didn't know you were out there, there would have been no need for this book.

ABOUT THE AUTHORS

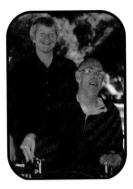

*Lydia Kelley &
Stewart Nordensson*

Stewart Nordensson has cerebral palsy, a disability often made more difficult because of public perception. People with CP are often pre-judged as retarded. For Stewart, one way to overcome this misconception has been through dog training. He has been training dogs for more than fifty years. He has exceptional insight into why dogs do what they do and how to train them — in obedience, service dog work, and correcting behavior problems.

That's why he wanted to write this book. He has read extensively in the area of dog training and behavior, discovering that virtually every book inferred that he could not train dogs for obedience or service dog work. He has proven over years of very successful training (several obedience degrees and four certified service dogs) that he can train his own dogs, and this book can teach you to train yours.

Lydia Kelley has been training dogs for almost twenty years and has been instructing classes in general obedience and service dog work. Lydia has always felt that understanding dogs is a key element in training, a factor frequently missing in basic obedience classes. Lydia has had several articles published in Off-Lead, a dog training magazine, and she has written extensively for TOP DOG.

Stewart and Lydia are founders of TOP DOG, a Tucson-based program that teaches people with disabilities to train their own dogs. This is where Stewart has been applying his unique and successful training methods for the past ten years. Now those methods have been put down on paper, so that you can benefit from his vast wealth of knowledge.

Using "teamwork," Stewart and Lydia have created this clearly written, easy to follow book. Stewart spoke his thoughts into the computer; Lydia took them, fleshed them out, and together they polished them. The result is a book which takes you step by step into the world of dog training and behavior, so that you can train your dog to whatever level you choose.

Stewart Nordensson, co-author of the Teamwork books died on October 5, 1999

PHOTOGRAPHS
(all photos listed from top to bottom)

Front Cover

- Tina Caracofe (juvenile rheumatoid arthritis) and Cora (border collie mix)

- John Cieslinski (multiple sclerosis) and Pepper (shepherd mix)

- Sandy Rider (Behcets) and Micah (golden retriever)

- John (degenerative disc disease) and Norma (lumbar fusion L4-5 & L5-S1) McKee and Magic (lab/rottweiler)

- Terri Roskey (multiple sclerosis) and Mazie (yellow lab)

Back Cover

- Mary George (rheumatoid arthritis) and Liberty (golden retriever)

- Linda Wilson (arthritis) and Jesse (black lab mix)

- Mike Landwehr (spina bifada) and Buddy (chow/newfoundland)

- Jim (chemical exposure) and Nancy (spinal stenosis/lupus) Martindale and Patch (jack russell puddin)

- Blake Gigli (spinal cord injury T12) and Bridgette (golden retriever)

TABLE OF CONTENTS

INTRODUCTION TO THE REVISED AND EXPANDED EDITION

Ten years ago, Stewart and I witnessed a dream come true—Teamwork was published. We had been working on it for several years, trying to make it the best possible training manual for people with disabilities. We knew that no book like it existed, and we knew that if we made it clear and easy to follow, there would be an audience for such a book. Ten years later, that's still true. Teamwork continues to help people with all kinds of disabilities learn the joy and satisfaction of training their own dogs as companions and helpmates.

Ten years is a long time, and many things change in the world, but a common sense approach to dog training is just as viable today as it was then. The way we teach the exercises in this manual is still the best way to teach them—using a positive approach, with lots of praise and food reward. Fads in dog training, as in everything else, come and go—people looking for a quick fix, an instant solution. But when the dust settles, it still comes down to patience, persistence, and positive attitude. So it wasn't that we needed to revamp the book or change the methodology—the basic principles are still very sound.

But even as the book went to publication ten years ago, we thought of things we should have included or things we could have worded better. So now, on the tenth anniversary of this excellent work, we present the revised and expanded edition to carry us into the new millennium.

There are two major changes. We added a chapter teaching the command "stand." This is a good command to teach your dog for many practical reasons, and it's especially important if you want to teach the "brace" command later. The other major change was separating "stay" into its own chapter. Both "sit" and "down" should be mastered before you begin to train "stay." We think this will make the progression of training much smoother.

*****

Stewart Nordensson died in 1999. He lived a valuable life. He never let his disability handicap him. He accomplished a great many things he could be proud of, but nothing pleased him more than seeing Teamwork, and then Teamwork II, in print. It was the culmination of his life's work—all his crazy, creative, and wonderful dog training ideas down on paper for all the world to learn from and enjoy.

When he passed away, I lost a good friend and supporter, in addition to my writing partner, and I still miss him. I felt his presence as I worked on these revisions. He was the inspiration for the founding of TOP DOG, and his memory continues to inspire those of us who knew him. His legacy, in these books and videos, continues to help and inspire people with disabilities all around the world. I think he would be pleased with the changes and additions to our book.

Lydia Kelley
May 27, 2007

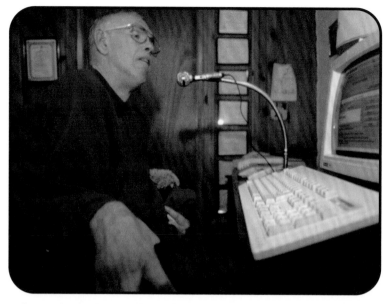

Stewart beginning to write the book, Teamwork, using DragonDictate®.

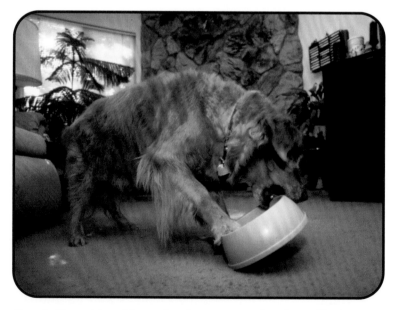

Sage (golden retriever) learned on her own to use her foot to flip the bowl
to give to her owner.

CHAPTER 1

GETTING STARTED
How to Use this Book Effectively

Humans have the ability to learn how to learn. Many animals also have this ability to some degree. When we work with our dogs diligently, they seem to learn faster and faster and, in some cases, can problem-solve. Because bending is difficult for Mary, she taught her dog, Sage, to pick up her food bowl after each meal. It was sometimes hard for Sage to grip the slippery top edge of the bowl, so Mary would flip the bowl over with her foot. Sage watched that a few times and seemed to think, "Well, I can do that." Without being taught, Sage used her foot to flip the bowl so she could take it easily in her mouth and give it to Mary. This is the result of a person and a dog learning to work together as a team.

This manual is designed to teach people with disabilities to train their own dogs. All previous training books have assumed that the trainer has certain physical abilities, that walking, talking, and making corrections are not problems. For someone in a wheelchair, "start off on your left foot," (the basic command to someone beginning "heel") is an impossible concept. For those with muscle spasms or no strength in their arms, "make a quick, firm leash correction" is simply not possible. Does that mean that disabled people cannot train their own dogs? For many years, it would seem that has been the belief. Even as the idea of service dogs to assist people with physical disabilities becomes increasingly accepted, it's still primarily a concept of someone training the dog for the person with the disability. For many people with disabilities, that's the best way to go. But it's not the only way.

Stewart Nordensson was not the only disabled person to show a dog in obedience competition and prove it can be done. He was, however, one of few who believed that any person with any physical disability can train his or her own dog if he or she wants to. And he devoted much of his life to figuring out the best ways for that to happen. This book is the culmination of years of research, practical application, study, and thought. It's Stewart putting down on paper the ideas he came up with over the years, so that his knowledge can help other people with disabilities.

Although we tell you how to teach your dog the exercises in a particular way, we realize that you are unique. Our instructions may not all work in your individual circumstances, but this book certainly will help. You will learn concepts of training, and you will learn to adapt them to your specific abilities and needs.

If you are one who learns better visually, we recommend that you use the "Teamwork" video (available in VHS and DVD) in conjunction with this manual. The video demonstrates each exercise, so that you can watch how it's done. Again, you may not be able to do it exactly as shown, but it will give you good ideas to try.

DISABILITIES

Stewart had cerebral palsy. How it affected him is different from how others are affected by CP, and it is different from how someone is affected by arthritis, a spinal cord injury, or multiple sclerosis. In other words, disabilities vary greatly, and people with the same disability vary greatly. So there is not "one right way" for a disabled person to train a dog. Stewart spent years helping others with disabilities find the ways to train their dogs, so he didn't just write about how someone with CP can train a dog. This book can be used effectively by someone with muscular dystrophy, arthritis, polio, spina bifida, and numerous other physical disabilities. It can also be a wonderful basic training book whether or not you have a physical disability.

Dog training is a very individualized activity. You must approach it based on your temperament, your strengths, and your dog. In this book, we have individualized some exercises within four categories: (1) Ambulatory (for those who walk without aid); (2) Ambulatory with Devices (which includes crutches, canes, walkers, walking sticks, etc.); (3) Manual Wheelchair; and (4) Power Chair (which includes all types of electric wheelchairs and scooters). We realize that even within these categories there are significant variations, and we have tried to cover as many of the variables as possible.

For each exercise there are basic concepts for everyone to understand. Some exercises are then broken down into those four categories. You may, of course, read it all, but you'll probably want to turn to the section that applies directly to you. If you use crutches to help you walk, look at the section "Ambulatory with Devices." This goes into specifics on the best way for someone on crutches to teach a dog that exercise.

DOGS

Just as you are different from other people, so is your dog different from other dogs. Some are very intelligent, but difficult to train; some are highly motivated to learn. This has nothing to do with your disability, but rather with your dog as an individual and as a member of his breed. You can learn to train your dog, no matter his breed, his size, his temperament, his sex, or his age. All dogs are trainable to some degree, but some are easier to work with than others, and you may have to be very creative to motivate your dog. Don't, however, think he's too old or too small or too stupid.

We use the male gender in referring to your dog throughout this book. That does not imply a preference toward male dogs. Both sexes are equally trainable. A neutered dog, either male or female, is much easier to work with, less distracted, calmer, neater. But our use of "he" is for simplification only.

If you don't already have a dog, take some time to research different breeds to decide the best choice for your circumstances. If you're considering training to the level of service dog, make sure the dog you choose is big enough, strong enough, and calm enough for your needs. Some of the tasks you might ask your dog to perform include picking up large objects, pulling or pushing your wheelchair, bracing to help you up, and opening doors. These are only some of the service exercises, but they all require a medium-to-large, fairly strong dog. It would be difficult for a Chihuahua or a miniature poodle to help you up or pick up heavy items for you. Although they can certainly be trained in basic obedience to make them better companions, they are limited as service dogs.

Whatever dog you have, this book will help you understand him and train him to the level you choose.

ATTITUDE

We have stated that there isn't one right method to train a dog. We suggest ways to approach each exercise and encourage you to develop your own method. There is, however, one right attitude in training a dog, and that is a positive attitude.

That actually has two meanings here. You must be positive that you want to train your dog. It's a big job, and if you're doubtful going in, you're more likely to quit. But you can do it, so believe in yourself and believe in your dog. This positive attitude is vital to success.

The other meaning of positive attitude is that your approach to the actual training must be positive. There has always been a school of thought in dog training that the dog must be dominated, cowed, forced into submission, a belief that the only obedient dog is the dog afraid of its owner.

We strongly believe that the absolute opposite is true. The only truly obedient dog is the dog who obeys because he wants to. We have seen and heard of so many cases where harsh training has backfired on the owner. An animal backed into a corner will wait for his opportunity to lash out. This is sometimes where force-training leads. The dog that has learned to obey you because it's pleasant to do so is a happy, obedient companion. And if you're planning to take the step beyond, if you think you want a service dog, there must be a positive bond between you and your dog. A service dog needs to be "on"—ready to work—all the time, so it's important that he has the desire to work.

You must, therefore, train with a positive attitude. Most important, you must never hit your dog. We can't stress this strongly enough. It's not a correction he can understand. All it does is make your dog afraid of your hand and wary of you. You want your hands to always be symbols of love.

If you think of your dog as a potential partner, who just needs to be taught what's expected of him, then you're well on your way. The ideas in this book will help you find the ways to physically teach your dog and mentally understand him. You'll learn what Teamwork is all about.

One of the new trends in dog training is the "clicker" method of training. This involves clicking a devise to signal that the dog has done something correctly. This is a positive training method, and, when used correctly, can be quite effective. But many people with disabilities have trouble holding such a devise, let alone clicking it at the precise moment. So, we encourage you to use your verbal praise as you would a "clicker." Be quick and positive with your praise, and you'll accomplish the same goal.

SLOW IS FAST

Throughout this book, you will find those three little words, reminding you of one of our most important philosophies of dog training. If you rush your training, pushing your dog too hard, you build a sloppy foundation. Dogs need time to absorb what you're teaching them. It might take a hundred repetitions of an exercise for a dog to really know it. This is a lot of repetitions. If you practice four sits a day, it will take nearly a month for your dog to have it solidly in his brain. So if you move on to sit-stay after a week, and down-stay the next week, you're probably overloading him.

This isn't a race. There's no prize for finishing all the exercises in the shortest time. The reward is over the long haul. You want your dog to work for you for years and years. Why not take the months required to get the solid foundation for this lifetime of service?

For someone with a physical disability, slow and steady is the only way to go. Your disability may prevent you from making quick corrections. Traditional trainers will tell you that "timing is everything." You must make your correction quickly so the dog understands; you must give the food reward instantly so the dog makes the connection.

It may not be possible for you to do anything quickly. But consistency and patience are far more important than timing. And consistency will be an individual thing between you and your dog. Your dog will understand the correction, will make the connection with the reward if you work as patiently and consistently as is possible for you on each exercise. Most importantly, give your dog the chance to really understand each step before you move on.

The traditional way to train a dog was to teach the exercise, then wait for him to make a mistake so you could correct him. Our idea is to minimize the chances for him to make a mistake, to teach the exercise so thoroughly that he will always succeed, and therefore you can always praise him. Of course, it's not realistic to say your dog will never make a mistake. But if you progress slowly through each exercise, you will find that you will rarely have to correct your dog. He will understand what you're commanding, and he will do it correctly, because that's the way he was taught.

ONE STEP AT A TIME

This book is written in a specific sequence. We believe that you must have a fundamental understanding of your dog in order to be part of a team with him, and the first chapters will help you attain this level of understanding. Knowing a little more about how your dog thinks will help you in all aspects of living and working together. Whether this is your first dog or your tenth, or whether your dog has already been trained by someone else, you need to understand how to communicate, recognize behavior patterns, and anticipate problems. This is how a partnership is formed; this is how

Teamwork is achieved.

No one can truly know what a dog is thinking, but the more aware you become, the easier the training will be. So take the time to learn as much as you can before you begin training. It's important to teach the exercises in the order presented. You begin with "attention," "sit," and "down;" then work on "stay," before you progress to the moving exercises—"come" and "heel." Please give each step of each exercise the time it needs before going on to the next step. That foundation of control exercises is important to establish. You are teaching your dog more than "sit" and "down;" you're teaching him to respect and obey you; you're teaching him that you're in charge. Remember that your physical strength or lack of it makes no difference.

Read a whole chapter before you begin teaching an exercise. This gives you a better understanding of the total exercise. You must understand it before you can expect your dog to understand it. If you're confused, go back and read it again. Don't try to teach something you don't quite understand. You'll only confuse and frustrate your dog.

When you're ready to teach the exercise, go back to the beginning of the chapter and review each step as you teach it. Although you can read through all the steps in a few minutes, remember that you want to teach each step thoroughly before you move on. How long each step takes is up to you and your dog, but don't be surprised if some steps take weeks to master. Your consistency and patience are the most important factors. And remember: "slow is fast."

THE LEARNING PLATEAU

Every dog will hit plateaus at different points in the training. These are days when the exercises you've been practicing successfully for several weeks suddenly become difficult for your dog to complete. It's important for you to be aware of this so that you're not frustrated when your dog seems to forget everything you ever taught him. He hasn't really forgotten. It's just a stage he's going through.

When your dog hits a plateau, the best thing to do is to find one exercise that he can do, and practice that. If you have to go all the way back to the first stages of "sit," do so. Work very short sessions at this elementary level, achieving positive results for a few days. It's not his fault. He's not being deliberately disobedient. Some theorize that his brain is working overtime to store all he's learned in long-term memory, and he may be on overload for a few days. Whatever the reason, almost all dogs experience this seeming setback. The best part is that once you get past this mental block, most dogs learn at an accelerated rate.

So be prepared for days along the way when your dog just can't seem to remember what he's been taught, can't seem to learn anything new. It may happen more than once as you proceed through your training. Take it easy and work him through it gently and positively.

HAVE FUN

Training your dog is a serious matter. You want an obedient, confident partner. This is true whether your goal is a well-behaved friend at home or a certified service dog who will accompany you to work or school, into restaurants and theaters, even on airplanes.

Training should also be fun. It's a wonderful sharing time with your dog and should be approached seriously, but with a sense of humor. You can have a good time and still achieve great success. A large part of this comes from wanting to understand and appreciate your dog. He's a living, breathing, thinking creature, not a robot. Enjoy his uniqueness, accept his canine characteristics, work with, not against, his personality.

And have fun!

CHAPTER 2

APPROPRIATE PRAISE
The Critical Importance of Praising Your Dog

Practicing random recalls in class, Lydia was holding onto a very exuberant golden retriever named Bambi. Her owner, Bill, had gone only a few feet away but that was farther than Bambi could tolerate. She twisted and pulled unexpectedly and Lydia ended up face down on the floor. Bill quickly called and Bambi was right beside him in a flash. Amid much laughter, Lydia got up, dusted herself off, and reminded Bill, "Praise your dog."

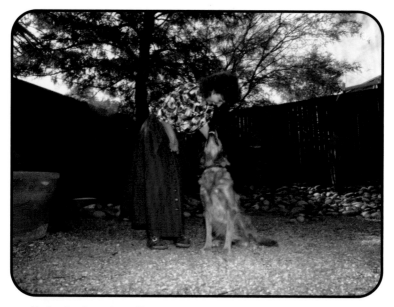

Enthusiastic praise will motivate your dog to work more quickly and happily. Mary George (rheumatoid arthritis) and Sedona (golden retriever)

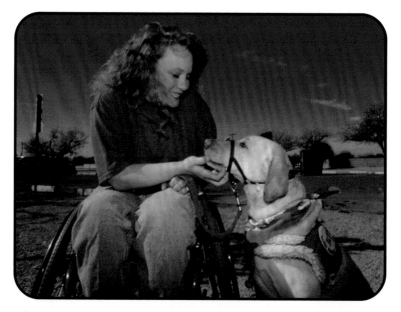

Appropriate praise may include a big smile and a scratch under the chin. Helen Enfield (spinal cord injury T 6-7) and Nutmeg (yellow lab)

WHY PRAISE?

Throughout this book, you will find the instruction to praise your dog. You need to understand praise—what it's for and why it's so important—before you can be expected to properly praise your dog. Some people cannot bring themselves to offer praise to anyone or anything. Perhaps they've not heard much praise themselves throughout their lives, so it's difficult for them to give it. On the other hand, some people praise their dogs all the time, using the same high-pitched tone whether they are pleased with their dogs or not. This praise loses all meaning.

Your goal is to create a team of person and dog working together, so you must learn to use positive training methods correctly. This will help you achieve your goal of Teamwork faster and more solidly than using negative training. The dog that works because he's afraid not to is not as calm, content, or creative. The dog that works with you as well as for you, because he knows there are positive consequences when he does what you command, is reliable and confident.

WHAT IS PRAISE?

Praising another human is generally different than praising a dog. When we compliment each other: "You look lovely tonight;" "That was a great speech you gave;" "What a beautiful painting," we are communicating almost exclusively with words. Our tone of voice doesn't change very much. We clearly don't sound angry, but we use the same tone as in normal conversation. If you tell your dog he looks lovely, and you say it in a normal conversational tone, he won't have any idea that you've given him praise. But if you get all bubbly and excited and say, "You're the ugliest thing I've ever seen," your dog will respond as if you complimented him. Words are not the key in praise; tone of voice is.

In the "Command" chapter (see page 61), we talk about your dog within his litter. The high-pitched happy sounds signaled play and joy. That's his conditioning, and it lasts his whole life. He will always associate that tone of voice with positives. He will also come to learn that certain words have a positive meaning, just as certain words have a negative meaning. But he won't know that instinctively. Your tone of voice when using the words will condition him.

Praise words should be easy for you to remember. Obviously, the easiest is "good." We automatically use the phrase "good dog" from the moment the dog comes into our home, so he quickly becomes conditioned by circumstances and tone of voice to know that "good" means good. It helps to use the command as part of praise, such as, "good sit," "good down," "good heel." You can simply say "good dog" after each exercise, but by saying the command word along with "good," it helps to reinforce the command. Praise can also be "thank you" or "attaboy!" Anything positive that is said in a happy tone of voice.

Praise doesn't have to be words at all. If you have speech difficulties, praise can simply be a sound in a higher tone. Or it can be a smile, a pat on the head, or even a rub with your foot. Whatever form praise takes, it needs to be something that feels positive to you and that is delivered when your dog does something you like. Your dog will come to understand it as praise. A nice side benefit to learning to praise your dog is that you can't be nervous or angry when you're praising. The very act of praising your dog relaxes you. The more you praise, the better you will become at praising.

WHAT IS APPROPRIATE PRAISE?

Appropriate praise will mean what is appropriate for you and your dog. The personality of your dog will often reflect the personality of you and your household. An active, outgoing person will generally have an active, outgoing dog. A quiet, reserved person will frequently have a calmer dog. So you may need to work on toning down or pumping up your praise.

It may be that your dog goes absolutely crazy whenever you say "good dog." You will then have to tone down your voice. An over stimulated dog will respond to a very quiet "good," or maybe a gentle touch on the head, or a simple smile. For this type of dog, keep your body as still as possible and your voice subdued. The dog that gets this excited can't concentrate on the lesson. Work very short sessions with very controlled praise, and then play ball or some other game with your dog to help burn off some of that energy and keep the associations positive.

On the other hand, your dog may be so laid back that he seems to be asleep half the time. He needs enthusiastic praise. You don't have to be loud; your dog will hear you just fine. But he needs a very spirited response from you when he does what you command. He needs to really know that you're pleased with him.

Remember that appropriate praise, whenever it appears in this book, will always mean appropriate to you. The most important thing is to be consistent in issuing the praise; always praise your dog when he obeys your command.

HOW TO GIVE PRAISE

Some people find praising is the most difficult part of dog training. They seem to be embarrassed and unable to praise. Praise really is the most important part of dog training. If it is difficult for you to praise your dog, you must work on it. This is the reward he is working for; this is the foundation of the bond between you and your dog. It's critical that you become able to give appropriate praise every time your dog deserves it.

Go in a room by yourself and practice. Work on a happy high-pitched tone of voice. Work on a smile. Think about the things that please you and say them out loud. Become aware of praising other people. You'll enjoy their response, and the practice will make you better with your dog.

You don't have to be loud or ridiculous. Simply get as much happiness and excitement in your voice as you can. Remember that this praise is your dog's reward, his paycheck. Don't have too much "withholding," or your dog will lose his enthusiasm for the work.

The opposite is also true. If every other word out of your mouth is "good dog," your dog is receiving too much "pay," and he is unable to make an association between a job well done and the praise. Praise given too often and at inappropriate times is not appropriate praise. It will only confuse your dog.

Each exercise will talk about the right time to give the appropriate praise. Your tone of voice should change from your command tone to a praise tone. It should be as enthusiastic as you can make it, based on your individual circumstances. Remember, "appropriate" means appropriate for you and your dog.

ALWAYS PRAISE

Praise will be our single most emphasized point. No matter what else you learn from this book, please learn to praise your dog every time he does what you want. Even when he has thoroughly learned the exercise and he does it successfully every time, he still needs to hear praise. The four hundredth time he sits on command should still be praised. If you stop the praise and think, "he knows I'm pleased with him," he may stop obeying as quickly; he may stop obeying altogether, because the incentive is gone. So, while you will taper off in the use of food, you must never discontinue the use of praise.

Praise will make your dog a willing, eager, happy partner, working for you because he wants to, because wonderful things happen when he does. A nice side benefit is that it makes the training experience much more pleasant for you as well. Both owner and dog are more relaxed, learn faster, and work better together.

CHAPTER 3

FOOD AS A TRAINING TOOL
The Importance and Correct Use of Reward

Using food to train a dog is a positive motivator. The dog enjoys learning because of the reward and that makes it more fun for the owner. Sometimes, though, a dog can become so focused on the treat that all else leaves his mind. Mary and Sedona had been working for several months and Sedona was becoming very proficient at various commands. But one morning her mind seemed to wander. She saw Mary pull out a treat and without waiting for a command, she sat, lay down, stood, gave her paw, lay down, and stood. Then, seeming to say, "Aren't I great, Mom," she sat expectantly waiting for her reward.

SHOULD YOU USE FOOD?

The answer is a resounding "Yes!" There is a school of thought that if you use food in training, you are "cheating" and creating a mindless stomach that will only work when food is around. But when food is used correctly, what you are creating is a positive, happy atmosphere for learning. It's not cheating to use food, any more than it's cheating to use a head halter (see Equipment, page 50). It's a positive tool to help accomplish an end result—a well-trained dog who works promptly and eagerly.

For someone with a severe disability, using food may be not only the quickest way to reach that end result, it may be the only way. You need to get and hold your dog's attention before you can begin to teach him anything (see "Attention" chapter). Food is the easiest way to encourage your dog to look at you. If you have no voice and/or no strength, food may be the only way.

If you have a strong aversion to using food in training, please examine that attitude. It may be symptomatic of a basic philosophy of needing to overpower your dog. We talked about positive attitude in the first chapter. Using food is part of that positive attitude. It's not the most important part—praise is most important—but food is a close second. If you think you don't know how to use food or perhaps you're not sure you'll be able to use food, this chapter will give you hints. But you may have to devise your own methods. Don't hesitate to experiment to find what works best for you.

"MY DOG GOES CRAZY WHENEVER FOOD IS AROUND"

Some dogs go completely out of control in the presence of food. This is a dog that jumps all over you and all around you as soon as he knows you have food in your hand. Obviously, if the dog is this much out of control, he cannot understand a command word and learn to obey it. You will have to condition him to settle down even when you have food. To do this, simply take a handful of his kibble and carry it in your pocket all the time.

Don't make a big deal of having food, and don't give any commands. This is a training exercise in and of itself. Don't take any food out of your pocket to give to him yet. Just carry it with you. Your dog will know you have it. In an hour or two, or a day or two, when he realizes he isn't going to get any, he will settle down. If he jumps all over you in hopes of getting the food, refer to the "Jumping Up" section in the "Behavior" chapter (page 36). You must correct this behavior, and condition your dog to be calm in the presence of food.

The first time you take a piece of food out of your pocket, expect your dog to go out of control again. Simply put the food back in your pocket and ignore the dog's begging. Correct any jumping-up behavior, but ignore everything else. It may take several days to condition a dog that gets this crazy over food, but if you are consistent, you can conquer the problem. You want to reach the point where you can take food out of your pocket without having your dog all over you. You want him under control. Once you reach that point, you will have a dog that will focus his undivided attention on you, so training becomes much easier.

THE CORRECT WAY TO USE FOOD

The secret to using food in training is knowing when to give it and when not to give it. It's not a matter of how fast you can deliver the treat. There are trainers who will tell you that timing is everything, and if you're too slow in your response to your dog, he will not be able to associate the reward with the action. That's not true. Timing is important. It's wonderful if you're able to give the food quickly. However, even if you cannot give the treat immediately, your dog will learn that the food is coming after a certain action, and you will get the same response. Your dog becomes used to your pace. He will still learn that there is a reward coming for the action.

The proper timing in the use of food is not so much how quickly it can be delivered, but rather that it follows appropriate praise. We talked about the importance of praise in the previous chapter. Be sure you read and understand its use. You must learn to use the praise and food together. You always praise your dog immediately for the action, and then give him the food reward.

After your dog knows an exercise, you can begin to taper off in the use of food rewards for that exercise. That means give him a treat every other time, then every third time, then randomly. Randomly means that you give him the treat sometimes, and sometimes you

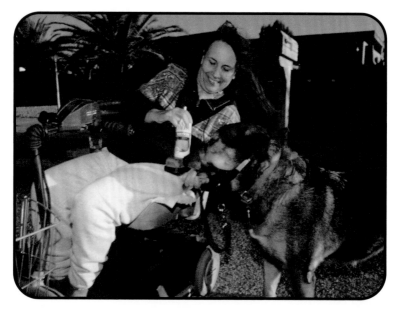

You can be very creative in the food reward you choose. Cheese squirted from a can is a delicious treat. Annette Stone (multiple sclerosis) and Bandit (shepherd mix)

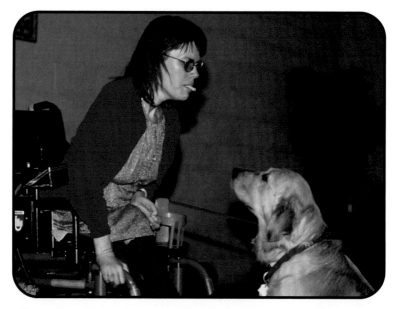

If you are unable to give your dog food from your hands, one alternative is holding the treat in your mouth. Roxie Meck (muscular dystrophy) and Angel (golden retriever)

don't. You want him always to think there might be food in it for him, but he will never know if this is the time or not. It keeps him interested. Never stop giving food all of a sudden. Your dog will stop paying attention. So always taper off and keep your dog on his toes. And always continue to lavish appropriate praise on your dog every time he obeys your command.

WHAT FOOD TO USE

If you have a dog that likes all food and will work for anything, then simply use his regular dry dog food. This is small, easy to carry, easy to handle. If your dog is finicky, you may need to find something that appeals to him—cheese, hot dogs, dried liver, beef jerky.

Food should be in small pieces. It must be easy to swallow so your dog only has to think about what he's being told to do. It takes too long for a dog to get through a big dog biscuit. You can't expect him to listen and obey commands while he's concentrating on eating.

Cheese is a wonderful food to use. Most dogs love cheese; it's soft and can be broken into small pieces. You can even use the kind that squirts out of a container, putting it on your finger or directly into the dog's mouth. Hot dogs, cut into small pieces, are also a wonderful reward. They may be a little messy, but that's a small price to pay for success. You can dry the hot dogs to make them easier to handle. Cut them into small pieces, then microwave them for about six minutes.

You may have to experiment to find the food that works best for you and your dog.

HOW TO GIVE FOOD

If you are able to hold the food in your hand, that's the best way. You will learn the timing within each exercise. Generally, as soon as your dog obeys your command, you give appropriate praise and then give the food reward. As you begin to teach each exercise, you will use food every single time. Don't give a command in the early stages of training unless you have food treats ready. Always praise first, then give the food reward.

If your dog tends to nip your fingers as he takes the treat, pull your hand away slowly and say "easy" or "gentle." If you pull away fast,

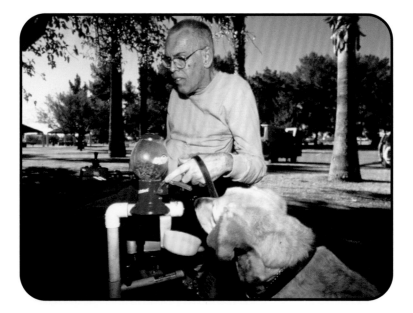

The gumball machine adaptation. Stewart Nordensson (cerebral palsy) and
Laura (yellow lab)

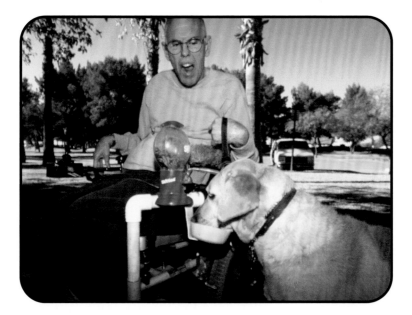

he will jump after the food. Close your fingers around the treat, if you can, and offer the treat again while saying "easy." Don't give him the treat when he's nipping. As soon as he stops nipping, say "good easy," open your fingers and let him have the treat. This may take several repetitions before he realizes that he won't get the treat until he's calm, but it's important for you to maintain this control.

If you are not able to hold the food, you may still be able to devise a means of giving your dog the reward. A piece of food held in a small cup will work if you're able to hold the cup. You can place a piece of food at the edge of a table and sweep it off to your dog when he has obeyed your command. You might hold the treat in your mouth and either spit it out to your dog or let him take it from between your teeth. These methods may take longer because your dog may be distracted by the logistics of getting the food, but he will make the association between the action and the reward. Try different ways of holding and giving food, and try different kinds of food. You might not be able to hold a piece of dry dog food but might be able to dip a finger in soft cheese and then allow your dog to lick that off. You need to evaluate your situation before you begin training and be willing to experiment as you go along.

Stewart adapted a gumball machine to fit onto his wheelchair. When he pressed the handle, food would fall into the bowl. The only thing you need to guard against is the clever dog that learns how to dispense the food whenever he wants! Be creative and use your imagination.

It may be that you will need someone else to dispense the food reward for you. This is a last resort if you truly cannot find any way to give the treat yourself. You must train this person to give food at the appropriate time. If you do have to involve another person, it's even more critical that appropriate praise comes from you before your dog gets the food. You might teach your friend to put the treat on your lap or your hand at the appropriate time. If your friend gives your dog his treat, you must repeat the praise, so he associates you with the reward. Your friend should stand as close to you as humanly possible so that the food can seem to come from you, and should not say or do anything distracting until your dog has completed the exercise.

BONDING THROUGH FOOD

Dogs are descended from wolves. Wolves probably first became domesticated when man gave the wolf scraps to eat. Instead of having to hunt game and frequently fail to bring it down, the wolf was offered an easy meal. He accepted and began to trust the one who provided for him. Thus the bond was formed, and food was the glue.

Food is not only the treats you give your dog during training. It's also his breakfast and supper. If you personally feed your dog his meals, his bond to you is that much stronger. Perhaps you don't feel that you are physically able to feed your dog, and you let someone do that for you. Even if you must have someone else do the actual feeding, you must be present in the room when your dog is fed. You should talk to your dog, and when the bowl is put on the floor, you should give a command to eat. All communication should come from you, and you should remain close to your dog while he's eating. This is why it's not recommended to use "self-feeding." If your dog can choose when to eat and how much, he doesn't feel any dependence on you. It may be more convenient to leave the food out, but it won't help your training or bonding. Feeding bowls should be put away after meals. They should not be visible unless you are there.

There may be ways that you can do more of the feeding for yourself than you ever thought possible. If you're in a wheelchair, you might get someone to put the food into a pail with a handle while you talk to your dog. You or your helper can then place the pail handle over some part of your wheelchair, and you can give your dog permission to eat. If you're ambulatory but can't bend down to the ground, place the pail on a stand.

You might try keeping food in a large bowl in a closet with a secure door. When you decide it's feeding time, you can open the door and give your dog a command to eat. Time the dog, depending on his size and appetite. When time is up, give a command to stop, and close the door. At first, you may need help closing the door, but your dog will learn the system.

Remember not to overfeed your dog. When you use food rewards

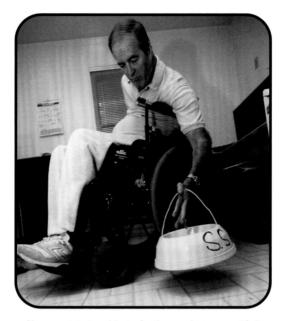

You want to be able to feed your dog yourself. A
handle attached to the bowl may make this possible.
Doug Somerville (spinal cord injury C 5-6)

in your training, give your dog a little less supper. It's not healthy for
a dog to be overweight. But never do you want to starve your dog
so he'll work more readily for treats. If your dog seems somewhat
indifferent to the food reward, use a different treat; find something
that does appeal to him. Change the time of your training session.
Don't train right after a meal. Instead, have a training session,
including food treats, just before his regular mealtime. Then feed
him a little bit less. Food is a positive motivator and should always
be used in a positive way.

In whatever feeding system you devise, try to keep feeding times
the same every day. Your dog needs a routine he can count on. It
helps to promote bowel movements at regular times, which is a big
help with a service dog. Plus, anything you do to make it clear to
your dog that he is dependent on you for his most basic needs will
help in both bonding and training.

CHAPTER 4

BEHAVIOR
Understanding Your Dog; Looking at Some Problems

Tom was a dog trainer, author, and AKC obedience judge. He had just judged at a large dog show, and the dog who took "high in trial" belonged to a friend. It had been a nearly flawless performance in the show ring with Rex losing only half a point in all the obedience exercises. That evening Tom went to his friend's house for dinner. When he rang the doorbell, he heard this nearly perfect obedience dog barking uncontrollably and lunging at the door. Over the din his friend called, "Wait until I lock Rex up in the basement." Tom had to wonder where Rex's perfect manners had gone.

UNDERSTANDING YOUR DOG

As humans, we tend to look at all behavior in human terms. But dogs are not human, and they do not react to situations in a human way, so it's important that you take some time to understand dog behavior. This will help in your day-to-day interaction with your dog, and will also improve your training skills.

This chapter will cover some general areas of canine behavior as well as some actions that we might consider problems. Dogs need to be taught what behaviors are acceptable and those that are not. You don't want your dog to be simply obedient; you want him to be well-mannered.

This book isn't intended to cover every dog behavior problem that might arise. There are many good books on this subject—some of them are listed at the end of this chapter—and we encourage you to consult them if problems come up that you can't handle. Simply by working with your dog and training him in basic obedience, you may find that many problems disappear. You also need to realize that so-called "problem" behavior is quite natural behavior to your dog. It becomes a problem only because it conflicts with your lifestyle. Then it has to be stopped or redirected. First, however, let's try to understand a little bit about the way dogs think and communicate.

PACK RELATIONSHIP

Because dogs are descended from wolves, they get their instinctive point of view from wolf behavior. Wolves live in packs, sometimes fairly large groups, with a social structure that is clearly understood by all members. Some are naturally more dominant than others. The leader, or leaders, is so easily recognized by the rest of the pack that a mere glance from a distance will cause others to crouch in submission. On the occasion when a dominant wolf is challenged, the ensuing scuffle is usually very brief. The weaker of the two will roll over on his back, exposing his belly and throat. The dominant one will hold the other in place for a few seconds before letting him go. There is no retaliation, no revenge. It's over.

This is a very simplified account of a complex subject. Books have been written on wolf behavior and studies continue. The thing that's important for you to understand is that your dog considers himself a pack member. Even if it's only you and your dog in your household, you are a pack. That means there must be a pack leader, and that must be you. If you are unwilling or unable to assume the role of pack leader, your dog will.

Does that mean you have to fight your dog and put him on his back? Absolutely not. Remember that the dominant wolf is able to control the pack with a look. Unless you own a dog with a very dominant personality, your dog will accept you as pack leader if you are fair and consistent in the way you deal with him. Perhaps your dog has been acting as pack leader because you haven't been. Once you start to train him to obey your rules and commands, most dogs will willingly relinquish leadership. If you find that he growls at you as you start to assert yourself, please consult a dog behaviorist in your area. Try to find one who understands dogs and doesn't feel the need to hit and abuse. That will not help in the case of a dominant dog; it will only aggravate the problem. If you approach training in a gentle but confident manner, as described in this book, your dog will probably be more than willing to turn authority over to you. It's a tough job being pack leader and most dogs aren't cut out for it. They've taken on the job simply because somebody had to do it.

Understanding this pack mentality can help you understand many situations that arise with your dog. We can never totally know what a dog is thinking, but if we recognize the deep-seeded instincts that shape the dog, we can come a lot closer.

BREED CHARACTERISTICS

After man domesticated the dog, he began to find many uses for this versatile companion. Over time he realized that he could select specific characteristics through breeding, thus creating animals with very different physical and mental attributes. Thus, although the beagle and the St. Bernard are both descended from the wolf, they lead very distinct lives today.

What your dog was bred to do can be a very important factor in your training. It is helpful to have some knowledge of the breed characteristics. We don't have the space to talk about every breed here, but you should take the time to find out about your own breed from a wide variety of available books. Talk to breeders. Contact the American Kennel Club. Check breed sites online. Find out as much as you can about what your dog was bred to do.

This is true even if your dog is a mixed breed. Try to determine what breeds make up your dog and learn about them. Your dog may have physical characteristics of one breed and mental characteristics of another. But just that little extra knowledge may help you understand why your dog behaves the way he does. Then you can stop fighting his instincts and begin to work with him as a teammate.

BODY LANGUAGE

Dogs communicate in several ways. Of course, they bark. If you listen to your dog you can recognize different barks for different situations—the happy bark for someone they know, the high-pitched bark of anxiety, the deep threatening bark for the garbage truck or the UPS man. There are also a whole range of whines, yips, and growls.

The primary way dogs communicate with each other is with body language. They also talk to us with their bodies, but most people don't appreciate the subtle signals. So take some time to watch your own dog and other dogs, and come to recognize what dogs are saying.

There are certain body movements that will indicate when a dog is happy and wants to play. His tail will wag. His face becomes open, almost laughing; you can see it in his eyes and mouth. He may pant in excitement and paw at you. The ultimate invitation is the "play bow." This is the position with the front feet stretched straight out, the rear end up in the air with tail waving above.

But you should also realize that a dog may pant from anxiety. He may paw at you in dominance. You need to try to catch all the signals from his body before you can be sure what he means.

A dominant or aggressive dog will raise his hackles and curl his lip. He will lean forward and stiffen, actually puff himself up, make himself bigger. The dominant dog will lean over the shoulder of another dog, putting himself in the top position. But dogs will also play this way. A curled lip might be a smile; hackles might be up from excitement. Again, put all the clues together before you decide what the dog is communicating.

A submissive dog will tuck his tail. His ears are back and his head is low. It's the opposite of the dominant dog trying to make himself bigger; the submissive dog tries to make himself smaller. He may put his head right on the ground as he approaches; he may go "belly up," lying on his back, exposing his neck and tummy; he may be so fearful that he urinates.

Your reaction to these signals is important. If you yell at your submissive dog for urinating as he greets you, it only increases the fear and prolongs the urination. Greeting this type of dog should be extremely low key, with no excitement at all. You should try not to lean over your dog—a very submissive dog sees this as a threat, which will only increase his tendency to urinate. Pat this dog under the chin, rather than on top of the head.

Most dogs will outgrow the submissive urination, although they may always approach you with head lowered and eyes subdued. If you gruffly tell that dog to get his head up, it only aggravates the fear. Understand that you have a submissive dog; try to keep your voice high and happy and all your interactions positive.

Taking time to learn your dog's body language will make training much easier. You will come to recognize when your dog's attention has wandered by the signals his body gives off—pricking his ears, stiffening up, wrinkling his brow. And you can interrupt your dog's actions before they begin. That way you won't have to correct him at all; you simply transfer his interest to something more acceptable.

TRANSFERENCE

Many behavior problems are easily solved or avoided by teaching your dog to transfer. If your dog has developed a bad habit— bothering company, for instance—you can teach him to substitute an acceptable activity. When company comes, get out your dog's favorite toy and begin playing with it, keeping it away from your dog while you both ignore the guests. After a few seconds, when your dog is very interested in his toy, give it to him and praise him enthusiastically for playing. It may only distract him for a brief period, but if you do this every time company comes, your dog may start associating their arrival with playing with the toy and begin to play on his own. You must get your guests to cooperate. They must ignore your dog, even if he brings the toy to them. Once your dog is older, more settled, and less annoying, visitors will be able to play with him. But during the early transference stage, they must help by ignoring him.

If your dog is chewing on something unacceptable, don't yell and rip the object out of his mouth. If you want him to retrieve things later, you must be careful not to make it a negative experience now. Again, begin to play with a favorite toy. When your dog comes over to investigate, calmly remove the object he was chewing on and say "no chew." Then substitute the toy and praise profusely.

Barking may be reduced through a combination of transference and correction. Think about your dog as a member of a pack. When one pack member barks at something, others frequently join in. This is pleasant and reassuring. When your dog barks and you yell and scream at him to stop, you have joined in. For your dog it's very rewarding to have the pack leader participate in the barking, so the noise will actually escalate. You yell louder and your dog barks more.

The first thing you should do is see what your dog is barking at. Some dogs bark at nothing, but you owe it to your dog to check out the situation. In time, you will recognize by the tone when he is barking at something serious.

Once you've evaluated the situation, you want to do something that will distract your dog and disrupt the pattern. Banging a garbage can lid or hitting a table will cause your dog to stop and look at the new noise. If your dog is afraid of loud noises, you can use a quieter tapping or whistle to get his attention. Use a command, such as "quiet," then praise softly, "good quiet." If the barking begins again, make the noise again, use the command again, then praise for the quiet. An aluminum can with some pebbles in it, called a "shake can," makes a very distinct and disturbing sound. Shake it behind your dog, or toss it near him (never at him). Most (but not all) dogs respond to this noise and stop what they were doing. As soon as he stops barking, praise for the quiet.

After you interrupt the barking with the noise and praise for the quiet, then you want to transfer your dog's attention to something acceptable. Use a favorite toy or food to get him to come to you. If your dog likes to play ball or retrieve things, you will probably soon have him fetching his toy as soon as you command "quiet."

Digging may also be reduced through a combination of methods, including transference. If your dog is a digger, your best bet is to allow him one place where he can dig. Any time you catch him digging where you don't want him to, tell him "no dig," then take him to the acceptable spot. Dig there yourself, if you're able. Praise him if he begins to dig there. If you don't catch him in the act, cover the undesirable hole with a board or block. You may have a yard full of blocks before he gets the idea. But if that one spot is the only place not covered, he'll dig there. You'll gradually be able to uncover the other spots. You might also try using a commercial "repel" product on the unacceptable places. Be sure to use such products carefully, always following safety directions.

Understanding what your dog was bred for may help you cope with some of these behaviors. A terrier is bred to "go to ground," so he will naturally want to dig. A retriever is bred to put things in his mouth, so he's apt to carry things around and possibly chew them. Watchdogs are more prone to barking. Work positively to curb these behaviors.

USE OF A CRATE

Some behavior problems can be alleviated with the correct use of a crate. There has always been a debate about putting dogs into crates. Some say it's natural for them to seek a "den," and that's why they go under tables and desks. But used improperly, as punishment or simply to get the dog out of the way, a crate becomes a prison.

A crate should be a place your dog feels safe. It must be comfortable, large enough for him to stand and turn around, with blankets or towels padding the bottom.

Your dog should be introduced to the crate gradually with lots of positive reward. Feed him in the crate; throw dog treats in and praise when he goes in after them. Close him in the crate for very short periods of time to get him used to it. If he barks and whines, ignore him. Praise when he's quiet.

Once a dog gets used to a crate, it will become his safe haven. If you think it's cruel to put a dog in a cage, think about putting a baby in a playpen. You do it so you can get a break and so the baby is safe from harming himself or your possessions.

If you leave your dog in a crate when you have to go out, he will not be able to chew your shoes or the couch. He will not be out in the backyard barking or digging. But you should have your dog out with you when you're at home. It doesn't help you bond with your dog if he's locked in his crate in another room.

Don't crate your dog for an excessive length of time. Dogs need exercise and changes of scenery and can develop physical and/or behavioral problems if the crate is too small or they are confined for too long.

Use a crate wisely and it can help you overcome many problems. Your dog won't develop bad habits, and in time you may be able to give him the run of the house. Then you can simply leave the crate there, and your dog may use it for his bedroom and his sanctuary.

SEPARATION ANXIETY

Because dogs are pack animals, it isn't natural for them to be alone all the time. They are social animals. Interacting with other living creatures is in their nature. It doesn't have to be other dogs; it can include cats, birds, and it certainly includes you.

When you leave home, your dog can become anxious. Especially at first, he doesn't know if you will ever return. Some dogs respond more strongly to this anxiety than others. The most common ways that dogs express this are with barking and chewing.

When you come home and find something chewed up, your natural reaction is to yell at your dog, but he doesn't even remember chewing. He's happy to see you, and you respond by scolding and yelling. He will have a negative reaction to your arrival and may learn to shy away from you when you come home. That doesn't mean he knows he "did something wrong." It only means he's learned that it's dangerous to be around you when you first come home. This might result in anxiety at your leaving and at your returning.

The first thing that you need to control is your temper. Your dog will learn to be by himself, and he will learn to stop chewing things, but it won't happen all in one day. Understand that some things might get destroyed. Remove your favorite things and anything dangerous to the dog. Be prepared to be calm, relaxed, and positive when you come home, no matter what chaos you find.

You want to make your leaving and returning as easy as possible on your dog. Always say the same thing as you go out the door. Just come up with a phrase: "I'll be right back; be a good dog;" "You have to wait right here;" "Guard the house." It doesn't matter what you say, but try to say the same thing every time. Say it in a calm, conversational tone of voice. Don't sound sad that your poor dog has to be all alone—that tone will increase his anxiety. Don't get excited. Just be matter-of-fact.

Follow the same process when you return. Greet your dog warmly and calmly, even if you can see he's chewed up your favorite pillow. Speak to him in a happy, relaxed tone of voice and pet him quietly. With some dogs, it's better not to say anything at all for a few minutes. Just come in the house, go to the kitchen, and have him sit for a treat. Then you can praise him and pet him.

Most of the damage is probably done in the first half hour after you leave, so you want to cover this period of high anxiety. Begin by leaving your dog for only a few minutes. Just walk away from the door, then come back into the house. Remember to say your leaving phrase as you go, but don't lock the door because you want to try to sneak back in. If you see your dog chewing something, you can scold him. Very firmly say, "What did you do? Bad!" Never hit your dog; use your tone of voice and/or a look to convey extreme displeasure. If you're unable to speak, you can bang the door or the wall, or toss the shake can.

As soon as your dog drops what he was chewing, you must stop correcting. If he comes to you, praise him quietly. Then act as if nothing has happened. Just go into your returning home sequence.

If you use an electric wheelchair or have trouble getting through your door, you probably will not be able to surprise your dog, so don't try. Just go away for short periods of time and then return. Vary the length of time you're away—one minute one time, five minutes the next, then two minutes, then twenty minutes. Do this over a period of several days so your dog gets used to your leaving and, more importantly, to your coming home.

There are some things you can do for your dog that may help relieve his anxiety. If he does get anxious, he needs something to chew, so provide chew toys for him. Anytime you catch him chewing anything inappropriate, scold him, gently take that object away, and give him one of his toys. Then praise him for taking the appropriate object. You're the pack leader and you decide what objects your dog can chew.

Never have more than two chew toys out at one time. If you have them scattered all over the house, you're essentially saying that he can chew anything he can find! Rotate the objects every few days so he doesn't get bored with the same ones. Some appropriate toys for your dog include nylabones, Kong toys, soft material toys, balls big enough that they can't be swallowed, and rubber toys (just be sure your dog doesn't remove the squeaker and swallow it).

You can increase your dog's enjoyment of these objects by sleeping with them. Not all at once, and be sure to warn your spouse! By keeping two or three objects near you all night, you put your scent on them. This helps your dog sense your presence when you're gone.

As you are leaving, drop one or two toys near your dog, say your goodbye phrase and leave. This will not insure that he will never chew anything of yours, but it may help.

Another way to give your dog a sense that you are still around is to take an article of your clothing (recently worn and not washed) and put it outside at the bottom of the door from which you leave. Do this in addition to rotating the toys. And consider leaving a radio on while you're gone. Tune it to the type of music you normally listen to, so that it's familiar to your dog and the house isn't totally silent. Always choose an FM station because a storm frequently causes static on an AM station.

During the early part of training, remember to keep things out of reach of your dog. Pens and glass cases left on the coffee table are too tempting for most dogs to resist. Put your shoes in the closet and shut the door. Don't leave enticing food on the counter, and keep the garbage out of reach. We go into detail in the "Leave It" chapter. You can teach your dog to leave food alone, but when you're not around, a roast on the table or chicken bones in the garbage are just too much to resist. Plan ahead and keep temptation from your dog.

These things, plus time and routine, should be enough to get your dog through his anxious moments. As he matures, he will naturally chew less. As you train him and his confidence grows, he will feel less distressed when alone. But be aware that changes in the home situation can cause a dog to revert to chewing and food stealing. If you go back to school or work, if you get married or divorced, try to guide your dog through the changes as sensitively as possible. Do your best to maintain your dog's routine—feeding, walks, companionship—or ease him into a new routine over a few days.

JUMPING UP

Breaking your dog from jumping up on people is one of the most difficult things to do, but it's critical that you accomplish it. Jumping can be dangerous to you and others, and it's unacceptable behavior in public.

Young, bouncy dogs tend to jump out of excitement, just wanting to be closer to you. Some dogs are trying to dominate when they jump on you. It means they have not totally accepted you as pack leader. Your normal reaction is to back up, but this just strengthens your dog's dominant position. If you are in a wheelchair, use the weight of the chair to help you. Simply move forward into your dog as he jumps. This will surprise him, and it returns you to the dominant position. If your dog jumps at you from behind, go backwards into him if you can. The idea isn't to run over your dog; it's to show him that you intend to be pack leader.

If you are steady on your feet, you can take a big step into your dog as he jumps. It should have the same effect as the wheelchair. But remember that you don't have the added strength and weight, so be careful. If you can use a piece of furniture to steady you, that may help.

As you move into your dog, command "Off!" in as deep and gruff a voice as you can manage. As soon as your dog's four feet are on the floor, praise, "good off." Don't be too enthusiastic in your praise or he will see that as an invitation to jump again. If he does jump right back on you, repeat the command, move forward and praise again when his feet hit the floor.

If you haven't the strength to do these things yourself, you may need help from a friend. Put your dog on leash and have your friend hold onto it. As you approach your dog, say "Off!" As he jumps, he will correct himself when he hits the end of the leash. Praise, "good off," as soon as he's on the floor.

This will take many repetitions. If your dog is young, exuberant, or dominant, jumping up may be a real problem, but you need to work consistently to bring it under control. That means you can't allow your dog to jump up sometimes and be petted and rewarded. You must make it an absolute rule that he is never permitted to jump on anyone. Later, when he's under good control, you may choose to teach him to jump up gently on your command. But on your command only. It's critical that your dog learns not to jump on you just because he wants to.

The same applies to jumping on others. Your dog may respect you as pack leader and not jump on you, but when guests come, he's all over them. You must get the cooperation of friends and family. Everyone must agree not to let your dog jump on them. If someone says, "Oh, I don't mind," you must say that you mind. You must explain how important it is to his training, and ask them to help you teach him.

When the doorbell rings, put your dog on leash before you open the door. Hold the leash firmly and command "Off!" as the visitor comes in. Keep your dog far enough away that he can't actually reach your guest, and each time he jumps, he hits the end of the leash and corrects himself. Don't get into a tug of war with your dog. You want slack in the leash so he makes a correction. Remember to praise every time all four feet are on the floor.

You might try transferring your dog's attention to something else, such as food or a toy. Refer to "Transference" earlier in this chapter.

If you don't have the strength to hold the leash and control your dog, enlist someone to help. You should stand close to your dog, and all verbal commands and praise should come from you. But your friend can make the leash corrections as needed.

If your dog knows and obeys the command "sit," give him a very firm command as the company comes in. He can't jump if he's sitting. However, this will only work if your dog thoroughly knows the sit command and obeys it promptly and completely. Without that total compliance, the desire to jump will cause him to disregard everything else. That will teach your dog to ignore the sit command. So unless you're sure he will obey, don't give any obedience command. Just teach him that jumping up is absolutely unacceptable and that he will never be rewarded for it.

As your dog learns what "off" means and begins to show some self control, anticipate him and give the "off" command before he jumps. You can see him start to jump, wanting to, but also wanting to obey your command. Then you can give enthusiastic praise and petting. Always, however, be ready for him to jump up again. Even after months of working on this, when he's settled down and hardly ever jumps up, you still need to give the command as he greets people. It's important to remind him that this command always applies.

FEAR

Some dogs are totally fearless while others are afraid of their shadows. Most dogs fall somewhere in between. Whether your dog has a lot of phobias or is only afraid of the vacuum cleaner, you need to condition him to face his fear. We will mention just a few anxieties here, but the general approach is the same no matter what your dog is afraid of.

An umbrella opening suddenly is disturbing to many dogs. Start with an open umbrella on the ground. Walk your dog around it and up to it and gauge his reaction. If he backs away from it, don't tell him, "it's okay." Talk to the umbrella in a high happy voice—it doesn't matter what you say; just keep chattering. Let your dog sniff it in his own time. As he approaches it, praise him. If he backs away, keep talking to him and move a little farther from the umbrella. Any time your dog moves toward it, praise him, but don't force him. That will only scare him more. Take as much time as you need simply to get your dog used to the umbrella lying quietly on the ground. Usually his reaction is because this is something new and different.

Once he's used to it, it won't be frightening.

When he's relaxed around the open umbrella, have a friend stand about ten feet away and slowly close and open it. Don't start with the sudden automatic opening; work up to it. That "pop" can startle any dog. If you get a reaction from your dog, have your friend move farther back. Have your dog on leash, but don't give him any commands—this is a training exercise in itself.

As your dog relaxes with the slow opening and closing, have your friend move in closer and closer. It should be a slow process—not all in one day. You can't rush overcoming fears; it takes time and patience. But it's important, especially for a service dog who will be accompanying you rain or shine.

When you can slowly open and close the umbrella in front of your dog, have your friend move back to ten feet away and this time pop the umbrella open. If your dog just has a normal startled reaction—flinching, standing up but not pulling back—praise him profusely. Any more serious reaction and your friend should move farther away. Work up very slowly to popping the umbrella open a few feet in front of your dog. Don't point it right at him. You want him used to the sound and the action; you don't need to torture him.

If your dog fears the vacuum cleaner, place it in the room where you feed your dog for a week or two. Then slowly move it closer to your dog's food bowl. Talk to the vacuum and pet it as you pass it by; otherwise, ignore it. Don't move it when your dog is around. When you actually use the vacuum cleaner, make sure your dog is outside or in another part of the house.

Then have someone turn on the vacuum while you and your dog are in another room. Talk to your dog and distract him. Praise him if he doesn't show any fear reaction. Slowly have the machine brought closer over a period of several weeks. Don't stress your dog. Always move the vacuum farther away if he becomes anxious.

If your dog is afraid of the car, you need to overcome this right now. Even if you don't plan to take him with you as a service dog, there are still trips to the vet, the groomer, etc. It's important that your dog be able to ride in the car without fear. Most dogs love to go in the car, and drives to the park or the woods become a wonderful shared experience.

At first, just walk around the car with your dog. Talk to him in a happy voice and give him treats. Next day, go out first and open one car door. Then walk with your dog around the car, again talking happily. Spend five or ten minutes a day by the car with a door open for several days. Move closer and closer to the car each day, unless your dog becomes anxious. If you chatter happily and distract him with treats, he should enjoy this time together.

When you're able to get up to the open door without an anxious reaction, the next step is to get him in the car. Use food and lots of praise. Toss a treat or a favorite toy into the car and if your dog jumps in after it, praise enthusiastically. Use a word like "car" or "in" as he jumps in, and another word, like "out" or "let's go" when he leaps out. Praise for both actions. Practice jumping in and out for several days, four or five times each day.

If he won't go in when you toss in a treat, have a friend hold him while you go to the other side of the car. Reach across with the toy or treat and encourage your dog to jump in, to come to you. Praise enthusiastically whenever he does it.

On very rare occasions a dog absolutely refuses to get in. You might need to lift your dog into the car or get a friend to. If you do this once or twice and have pleasant experiences in the car, your dog will probably begin to get in on his own. Some dogs, however, suffer from car sickness. One theory holds that static electricity is a major cause of car sickness. To remove the static, attach a leather strap to some metal part of the car and allow it to drag on the ground. If this doesn't help, consult your vet.

Fear of sudden or loud noises is a very common phobia—thunder and fireworks are the most typical. You can get a tape of these noises and play it at a distance, then move it closer as your dog gets used to the sound. But your dog may not consider this realistic. You can try to distract him during a thunderstorm by playing ball or working on obedience exercises in a happy manner. But the dog that is very afraid will not be able to concentrate on anything else. Turn on the TV or radio tuned to an FM station, as there may be static on an AM station during a storm. Close curtains—the darker you can make it, the more relaxed your dog may feel.

Whatever you do, don't tell your dog that it's okay. He doesn't understand that you mean it will be okay in a little while. He will assume that you approve of his fear reaction. If your dog just wants to lie in a closet quietly until it's over, let him. If he gets frenzied, consult your vet.

Don't try to flood a frightened dog with the sounds he fears—in other words, don't take a scared dog to a fireworks show. The only way to overcome the fear is to build up slowly, moving the dog closer to the sound when he shows no anxiety. The trouble is that thunderstorms come when they come; we have no control over them, and your dog will probably show fear before you have any idea that a storm is coming. Be alert. Try to be as upbeat and unafraid as you possibly can and convince your dog that there's nothing to fear.

REFERENCES

If any of these problems seems to be overwhelming, please refer to any of the books listed below or consult a behaviorist in your area. A good behaviorist will evaluate the situation and help you understand why it's happened and what can be done to correct it. He or she should not advocate hitting or excessive punishment or abuse. Pouring water in a hole your dog dug and then sticking his head in it will not teach your dog not to dig. And you should be leery of an "expert" who recommends such a correction. A good behaviorist works with you and teaches you how to work positively with your dog. Beware of the ones who want to take your dog to their facility. They may correct your dog's behavior while he's there, but it will not help when he comes home. You have to learn what to do yourself and when and how to do it, or the situation will continue.

Remember that many "problems" are simply a dog's way of trying to cope with a confusing situation. With time, patience, and training, many problems correct themselves.

BOOKS

There are several volumes available covering most dog breeds. Your library may have some or consult a pet shop or book store, and, of course, take advantage of all the internet has to offer. Read as much as you can about your dog's breed. It can really help you understand him.

For behavior, we recommend any of the following books to help you gain understanding and knowledge. Though some of them have been around for a while, they offer wonderful insight into canine behavior and how to live with it.

William Campbell
Behavior Problems in Dogs
Michael W. Fox
Understanding Your Dog
How to Be Your Dog's Best Friend
Karen Pryor
Lads Before the Wind
Don't Shoot the Dog
The Monks of New Skete
How to Be Your Dog's Best Friend
Cesar Millan
Cesar's Way
Suzanne Clothier
Bones Would Rain from the Sky

CHAPTER 5

EQUIPMENT
A Look at Various Tools to Help You Train Your Dog

One exercise in advanced obedience work requires a dog to jump over a high jump, retrieve a dumbbell, and then come back over the jump with the dumbbell in his mouth. To teach his dog this exercise, Stewart had Bev on a long line. This allowed him to maneuver his wheelchair around the jump and drop the dumbbell, then encourage Bev to come over the jump to retrieve it...he thought. Stewart was barely to the other side of the jump when Bev came flying over, landing squarely in Stewart's lap. No one was hurt, and the long line didn't even tangle.

TRAINING TOOLS

It is possible to train a dog without ever placing any piece of equipment on him, but it would probably take a very long time and an enormous amount of patience on the part of the trainer. So man has created an array of devices to help in the training process. What you prefer to work with is an individual choice. It may involve some trial and error on your part until you find the right tools for both you and your dog. We will discuss a few of the more common ones in this chapter, but be aware that there are many more out there, and you may discover something that works perfectly for you that we've never heard of. Or you might devise your own collar or leash that works better for you. Don't hesitate to use your imagination in finding the right tool.

Remember that training tools are just that. They are tools for training. Don't expect a miracle if you try some wonderful new kind of collar. Training still takes patience and consistency on your part.

Never leave any kind of training collar on your dog unattended. We will mention that again and again because it is such a dangerous practice. If the collar catches on something, your dog will pull away to free himself and might end up hurting himself or even choking to death.

COLLARS

Your dog should wear some type of buckle collar at all times. This should have his local license attached and perhaps some other form of identification, so that someone can notify you should he become lost. This collar should be snug enough that it won't slide off easily, but should not be tight. It can be flat leather, rolled leather, or nylon. Remember that this is a collar with a buckle, not a choke chain.

It may be possible for you to do all of your training using just this collar. In this manual, we show you how to teach the control exercises—"attention," "sit," "down," and "stay"—first. The primary training tools used for these exercises are praise and food. You teach your dog to listen to you; that there are positive rewards when he does. By the time you get to heeling, you will have your dog's attention, and very few leash corrections should be required.

But if you need more control, there are other tools available. You may want to try a "training collar" or a "head halter."

TRAINING COLLAR

The mainstay of obedience training has traditionally been the training collar, also called a choke collar. Those who use gentler training methods prefer to call it a training collar and encourage their students to learn to use it correctly, so it is only tight around the dog's neck for a second. It never chokes.

The training collar may be made out of metal with various size links, or nylon of various thicknesses. There are several advantages to metal. It releases better (we'll go into the importance of releasing below), and it makes noise when used correctly, as an added signal to the dog. Nylon is easier on a dog's coat, but if the collar is used correctly, it shouldn't be continuously pulling on the dog's coat anyway. It comes down to an individual choice. If you prefer the nylon and find it works for you, then that's what you should use.

PRINCIPLE OF THE TRAINING COLLAR

The idea behind the training collar is that you have a method of communication with your dog. It's not so you can pull him around with the collar continuously choking him. If someone pushes you, you have a tendency to push back. It's an instinct. If someone pulls on you, your tendency is to pull the opposite way. That's true for dogs, too. So if you use the collar and leash to pull on your dog, his instinct is to pull away. Dogs are strong, and if your disability makes you weak, your dog will win that contest.

The correct principle of the training collar is to keep the dog off balance. If someone pulls you when you don't expect it and immediately lets go, you'll be knocked off balance and won't have time to pull back. That's what you're doing with the "jerk and release" of the training collar. You're throwing your dog off balance only for a second. And he doesn't like that sensation anymore than you do. He will quickly learn to pay closer attention to you so that you can't surprise him.

The only correct way to use a training collar is with the "jerk and release." Its primary use is in heeling. If your dog pulls ahead, you use the leash to jerk the collar tight for a second and immediately release it. If you have made a good "correction" you will be able to hear a noise from the collar. And since a dog's hearing is seventeen to twenty-five times better than that of the average person, your dog will hear it too. If you keep the collar tight for more than one second, you have lost the advantage of surprise, and you're wasting time and effort. Worse, you might damage your dog's larynx. A correction must be followed immediately with praise. If you make the proper correction, your dog will stop pulling and will be beside you in the proper heel position. Then he must hear praise.

PUTTING THE COLLAR ON

The training collar has two equal size metal rings, one on each end. To make a loop, hold one ring in each hand between your thumb and forefinger. Lower one ring the length of the chain, then feed the chain through that ring until the two rings come together. Now you have a loop which you slip over your dog's head.

It's important that you put the collar on correctly. If you put it on incorrectly, the chain will not loosen even though you release it, and you won't be able to make a proper jerk and release correction.

Attach your lead to the "live" ring, the one without the chain through it. Have your dog sit beside you on the side you want him to be on. The chain attached to the leash should come across the top of his neck. If that length of chain is under the dog's neck, it won't release. Try it on your arm and see the difference. Then try it on your dog. Everyone puts the collar on backwards sometimes, but try to be aware that it goes on correctly each time or you won't be able to communicate with your dog.

When you put the training collar on, remove your dog's regular buckle collar. The extra collar may catch the training collar so that it won't release properly. After the training session, remove the training collar and put the regular collar back on.

CORRECT SIZE

Every good instructor will say that the size of the collar is critical to proper corrections. They will tell you that there should only be two-to-three inches of play. In other words, when the collar is tight around the dog's neck, there should never be more than two or three inches of extra chain.

It's true that it's much easier to get a quick correction when the training collar fits well. If it's easy for you to get the collar on and off your dog, you should choose one that goes easily over his head (not pinching his ears) and gives you that two-to-three inches of slack.

But what if it's difficult for you to put the collar on and off? What good is a well-fitting collar if you have to get someone else to put it on your dog for you? The point of teaching you how to train your own dog is for you to do all the work. In some cases, that's not possible. But if a way can be found for you to do it, then that's what we're striving for. You may be able to put a collar on by yourself if that collar is way too big.

Dianne is a quadriplegic with movement in her arms, limited movement in her hands, and no strength in either. She uses a collar that would send traditional obedience instructors running off screaming and tearing their hair. Her collar is the correct size for a large German shepherd, and she is working with a small malinois named Radar. Dianne makes the loop in her collar, then holds it in her hand to the side of the wheelchair. Radar puts his head into this oversized circle, and Dianne moves her hand back and drops the collar onto Radar's shoulders. The collar is way too big, but Dianne is able to take him for walks and train him when she otherwise couldn't have.

Pam has muscular dystrophy, no strength and very little movement in her arms. She was unable to use a traditional metal chain because she couldn't keep the loop. She uses a thick stiff nylon collar called a "mountain collar" several sizes too big for her dog. She also needs her dog to get closer to her in order to put on a collar. She taught her dog, Goofy, to put her front paws on Pam's wheelchair. Using food, she taught Goofy to put her head through the loop while Pam slipped it on over her ears.

In both cases, to remove the collar, the owner slips a finger under the collar and hangs on while the dog backs up. If the collar were not oversized, it would catch on the dog's ears and the owner might be unable to hang on with the finger.

The point is that if you have limited strength or dexterity in your arms or hands, an oversize collar might work perfectly for you.

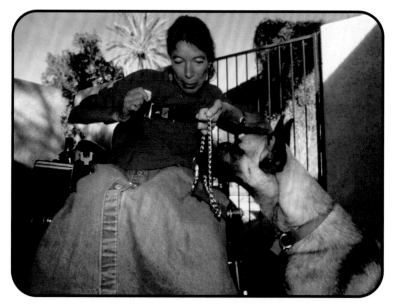

Using an oversized collar may be the only way for you to put the collar on
and off your dog. Food encourages your dog to put his head through the
loop. Dianne Kalal (spinal cord injury C 5-6) and Radar (Belgian malinois)

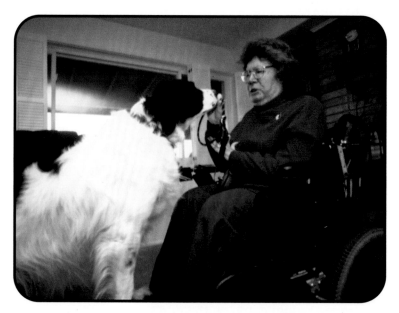

Sometimes it helps to have your dog get up on the wheelchair to get in and
out of his collar. Pam Rhatigan (spinal muscular atrophy)
and Goofy (border collie/Australian shepherd)

Don't worry if a traditional instructor tells you you'll never be able to make proper corrections. You may not make them to his satisfaction, but at least you'll be able to put on the training collar and work with your dog by yourself. And you will make corrections that your dog will learn to understand. A "proper" correction is simply a correction that works for you and your dog.

To train your dog to put on his collar, make a loop in the collar and hold it in front of him. Hold a piece of food on the other side of the loop or have a friend hold the food while you give the commands. As your dog goes for the food and thus puts his head through the loop, say "collar" and praise and give him the food. Since the loop is big and isn't a struggle for you or your dog, he will quickly learn that there's a reward for placing his head in this loop.

From a wheelchair, try holding the loop down beside you and teaching your dog to put his head into it or having your dog come up on the chair so his head is close to you. Always remember to give a command as your dog goes into the loop. He will learn to associate the word with the action. Again, always remember to reward your dog, verbally and then with food.

The easiest way to remove the collar, as Dianne and Pam found, is to hook a finger or two under the collar on top of your dog's neck. Pull forward gently but firmly and your dog will instinctively pull back. Again, because the collar is so big, it will slip over the ears without pinching. By holding the collar at the top, it will retain its loop without pulling tight. Use a different word, such as "back" and say it every time your dog comes out of the collar. He will come to associate the word with the action and will then pull back on his own.

It may take time to reach the point where your dog knows that he's supposed to move into and out of the collar, but if you approach it in a positive and patient manner, it should be something that he learns willingly. As your dog gets used to the action, you may be able to downsize the collar. Make sure you can still get the collar on and off easily by yourself. That's much more important than a "proper" fit.

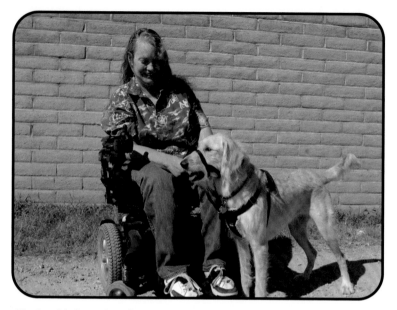

The head halter, when fit correctly, sits comfortably on the nose and allows a dog to fully open his mouth. Helen Enfield (spinal cord injury T 6-7) and Monet (labradoodle)

HEAD HALTER

The other major type of training collar isn't a collar at all. It's very much like the halter on a horse. There's a strap that goes behind the ears, a strap across the nose, and a ring under the chin where the leash attaches.

The usual response to seeing a dog in a head halter is to ask, "Is that a muzzle?" It is not a muzzle. It is not tight around the dog's mouth. The dog can open his mouth fully, can eat and drink and pick things up.

There are different brands of head halters. You may need to look at several before you find one that works for you. The fasteners are sometimes hard to work, so be sure to check that. However, you can easily change the fastener to one that you can manipulate better. The head halter, like the training collar, is a training tool. It is for training only and should never be left on your dog unattended.

PRINCIPLE OF THE HALTER

The principle of the head halter is that where the head goes, the body will follow. It's like power steering. It doesn't call for any kind of strength on your part. You don't make any kind of jerk and release; you just hold on. Your dog will make all the corrections himself. It might make the difference between you being able to walk your dog or not. But it still has to be used correctly for it to work, and it doesn't work for every dog.

There's an interesting reason why it doesn't always work. When a mother dog wants to discipline her puppies, one way she corrects them is to put her mouth gently over the puppy's muzzle. The puppy knows instinctively that he better stop what he's doing because Mom doesn't like it. The halter does the same thing. When the dog is out of position, the leash will tighten the strap across the dog's nose. This is a gentle reminder of Mom's correction. For a dominant dog, this is a very difficult thing to accept.

If you're lucky, you can put a halter on and immediately begin working with your dog. He may never object to it, just accept it like any collar. In other cases, no amount of gentle work and patience will ever get him to accept it. He may paw at it, rub his face on the floor and on you, twist, and pull. He can't concentrate on training or anything else except getting rid of the halter.

Most dogs fall somewhere in between. If you take some time at the beginning and introduce the halter in a gentle, positive way, you can usually avoid the complete protest. But expect some objection. The first time a puppy is walked on a leash with a regular collar, he bucks and pulls. It's something new and confusing. The halter is much more than that. There's a strap across the muzzle; there's something in front of the eyes. This takes some getting used to.

PROPER FIT

The fit of the halter is very important. If it's too small, it will be tight across the muzzle all the time and thus would make a correction on the dog just for opening his mouth. It will also be a struggle to get on and off. If it's too big, the nose strap will ride up into the dog's eyes causing discomfort and annoyance. The only way to get a perfect fit (and that's very elusive) is to take your dog with you to a store that carries a variety of halters and actually try them on. You might also consult your vet who might sell halters or be able to tell you where to get them.

Don't just grab your dog and force this apparatus on him. Remember that this is something very new and different and a little scary. Never come at your dog from the front with this "thing." Approach from the side, use a gentle and reassuring tone of voice, and have food ready to distract him. If you're being helped by a salesperson, be aware that your dog may already be wary of that person. Don't let the stranger force the halter on your dog if he seems resistant. Relax, use patience, praise your dog for each small step. Take the time to find the proper fitting halter, and all future steps will be easier.

USING A HALTER

The halter can be the easiest, perhaps the only, way for you to train your dog, but it must be used correctly. There's potential for abuse, possible spinal injury, and certainly for confusion. You must be sure you're giving the correct signals to your dog if you expect him to learn. Remember that the halter is for training only. Take it off after a training session and put it away, because your dog may find it irresistible to chew.

If your dog seems unsure about the halter, build up the association slowly and positively. At first, only touch his nose with the strap and do this several times to get him used to it. Give appropriate praise. To get him to put his nose through the strap, hold a piece of food just beyond the strap. Praise as your dog reaches for the food and puts his nose through. Do this several times without buckling the halter.

The first time you buckle it on, be sure to use both praise and a food reward to make a positive connection. If your dog doesn't object, you can leave the halter on for a few minutes. Don't attach the leash to it yet; the leash should be attached to his regular collar. If your dog begins pawing at the halter, distract him. Get him to look at you and praise him and give him a food treat. Don't give him food for pawing at the halter; the praise and food should come when he stops the pawing and looks at you. If the pawing becomes too frantic, move around with your dog to get his mind on something else. Then remove the halter. Don't remove the halter while he's pawing at it—you don't want him to think he can get it off that way.

Put on the halter just before you feed him and let him wear it while he eats. If he's more interested in getting rid of the halter than in eating his supper, it may be that the halter won't work for your dog. But most dogs come to accept the halter and eventually will ignore it.

For several days just put the halter on without the leash attached and let him wear it for short periods of time while you observe him. When you do attach the leash, work only for a minute or two, then attach the leash to the regular collar. Do this back and forth for several days to get your dog accustomed to the halter with leash attached. Then you can use the halter for all training.

Your attitude when using a halter is important. When your dog paws at this thing on his head, you will have a natural reaction of thinking, "He hates it." He doesn't hate it. He may not like what it does since it gives you control, but that's something he's just going to have to get used to. Don't get emotional and sympathize when he paws and rubs. Tell him "no rub" firmly and distract him. You will notice that he doesn't have to paw at it when you're giving him food or when he's sniffing a bush. Remember that you are the one in charge; you choose what your dog will wear.

If you're used to using a training collar and are now using a halter, concentrate on the proper way to make corrections. Don't ever jerk a halter. The training collar is used around a dog's neck where there are muscles and sometimes a thick coat. The halter is pulling on the dog's nose. If you jerk it, it can cause a whiplash effect.

Simply hold the leash firmly. Your dog will pull it tight if he's in the wrong position. When you gently tug in the direction you wish your dog to go, his head and body will come around.

The halter can be used to teach every exercise, and it may be the only way for you to work with your dog if you lack strength in your arms and hands. Your dog will come to associate the halter with "work time." He will know you have control of the situation.

The head halter may be a wonderful way to go, but if you are unable to put the halter on and off, it may not be the best tool for you. If you can put on a training collar but can't work the halter, the collar will be the better training tool simply because you can do it yourself. If you have to get help to put on any training device, it doesn't matter. Choose the one that works best for you and your dog, and accept help willingly in getting your dog ready to work. This book will help you find ways to augment the training tools, using your wheelchair or other devices, including, as always, praise and food.

LEASHES

Collars and halters are the means of communication and correction. What connects the collar to you is the leash, and there are several to choose from. You may want to own two or three kinds which you'll use in different situations.

The standard leash is made of leather or webbing. There are chain leashes, but we don't recommend them because they're hard on your hands. Leashes come in various lengths, with four-foot and six-foot being the norm in obedience training. There's a snap on one end which attaches to the collar or halter. There are different kinds of snaps, so find the one easiest for you to work. The other end of the leash has a loop which you hold in your hand or place over the handlebar of your wheelchair if necessary.

If a six-foot or even a four-foot leash is too much for you to handle, try a "traffic leash." This is only about two feet long, so there isn't extra leash to get caught in crutches or a wheelchair. It's a handy length when walking with your dog in crowded places, but there's no extra line to let your dog wander off to relieve himself.

Leashes come in varying widths as well as lengths. A thin leash may be hard on your hands. Leather may feel better than webbing, or vice versa. There are also leashes of thicker, softer webbing. Try several to see which works best for you.

Stewart developed his own leash system. On a six-foot leash, he attached a loop about a foot in from the snap. He put the loop at the end of the leash over the handle of his wheelchair, then placed his hand through the other loop to control his dog. If his hand slipped out of the loop, the leash was still securely attached. Double loop leashes, such as this, are now available in many catalogs and pet stores.

Samir was only nine when he began training his dog, Ravi. He needed a leash that he could loop over his shortened arm, so that,

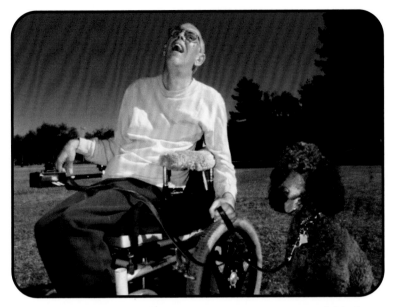

Stewart devised this double loop leash. It allows him to attach his dog securely to his wheelchair and hold a loop in his hand. Stewart Nordensson (cerebral palsy) and Maria (standard poodle)

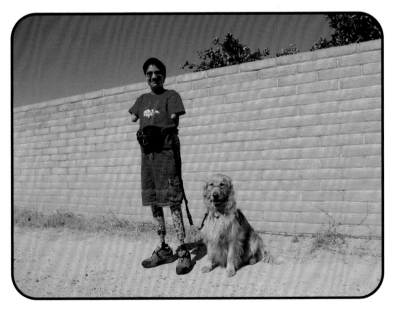

A hands-free leash may work well, as long as there's no danger of your dog pulling you over. Samir Madden (bilateral above elbow, bilateral below knee amputee) and Ravi (golden retriever)

even though he didn't have hands, he could still control Ravi. His mother actually made the leash, by sewing on a second loop, padding it, and adjusting it to fit snuggly on Sami's upper arm. Sami then put the rest of the leash over his other shoulder. This way, he could keep Ravi close to him and still be able to use his arms to hold a treat to direct Ravi as he taught each exercise. Now that Sami is older and stronger, he's using a hands-free leash, called the Buddy System, that attaches to a belt around his waist. For someone with no strength in hands or arms, this might be a good choice, as long as there's no danger of your dog pulling you over.

LONG LINE

A long line can be a very useful piece of equipment, both for training and everyday use. Stores and catalogs sell a variety of webbed lines, in lengths from ten to fifty feet.

During training, the long line is used primarily in recall so that you can get farther than six feet from your dog but still have control. If he chooses not to come to you, you can use the line to bring him in to you. You can also use it on the stay exercise. You can practice from greater distances but still have him on leash. It's much safer.

In everyday life, the long line is handy because it allows your dog a sense of freedom but gives you control. You can walk your dog and allow him to move more than six feet from you to relieve himself or just to sniff and explore.

FLEXI-LEASH

The retractable leash might be the perfect long line for you. This comes in different lengths and strengths. It has a plastic case (various colors are available) with a handle and a thumb button. Thin nylon line comes out of the case with a snap that attaches to your dog's collar. You can stop it by pressing the thumb button which puts a brake on the line. You can even lock it in place at any point. Release the brake and the line goes in or out with your dog. When your dog is coming toward you, the line retracts automatically so it doesn't get tangled. This can be a wonderful advantage.

You can try one to see if it's something that will work for you. See how it feels in your hand, and work the thumb button so you can decide how easy it is to use. It takes some practice for anyone to use a flexi-leash adeptly, but you should be able to tell right away if it's something your hands can manage.

Some people use the retractable leash as their only leash. They lock it in place at the proper length for walking with their dog, then let it out whenever they need more. It can be a great advantage to have any length of leash you might require in one system. But the plastic case is big and may feel awkward, and the line is thin and can burn. You are the only one who can decide if it's the right leash for you.

Keep all equipment where your dog can't chew it. They seem to be very tempted to chew their leashes, collars, and halters. So put them all out of reach when you're not using them.

ATTACHMENTS TO YOUR WHEELCHAIR

In order to work with your dog from a wheelchair you may have to devise a method of attaching him to your chair. If you haven't the strength to hold onto the leash, you need to have your chair hold the leash for you. The simplest way is to put the end loop over your chair handle, arm rest, or brakes. Then perhaps you can put a second loop in the leash which you can hold onto. If you can manage it, it's better if you are able to touch the leash, at least some of the time. Much of the communication between you and your dog goes directly through the leash, and your wheelchair is not able to communicate the same way you can.

If that's not possible, then you may want a system of changing from a short leash for heeling to a longer leash to allow your dog to lie down. One thing that seems to work quite well is to attach a carabineer, a link used in climbing, to your chair. These are available in hardware and sporting-goods stores. It allows you to push the leash through the link at whatever length you need. There are other optional attachments available; don't hesitate to experiment to find the system that works best for you.

CAUTION

Be aware that if you attach your leash permanently to your wheelchair, you cannot let go of your dog in an emergency. This may simply have to be the price you pay, but you need to be alert. In the situation of a strange dog attacking you, your only recourse is to use your chair as an offensive weapon. Try moving your chair quickly into the aggressive dog if possible. Your goal is to protect yourself and your dog. If the hostile dog bites your wheelchair, he probably won't bite anything ever again. Though very difficult, it's important to remain calm. You especially don't want to yell, as that only excites both dogs. This is a very scary situation, but if you can remain calm and confident and move forward as fast as possible, this is a dominant act and most dogs will retreat.

If you have the ability to release your dog in a situation like this, that usually solves the problem. Two dogs, without human interference, will generally greet each other and very rarely fight. But if you need to have your dog attached to your chair, you just have to be aware, alert, and prepared for every predicament. Above all, try to maintain a confident air. Dogs sense fear, and fear is the one thing you don't want to project.

CONCLUSION

Equipment is very important in training, as you have now learned. Whatever collar and leash you decide to use should always fit properly and be of good quality. Training collars are quite inexpensive. Don't buy a cheap supermarket brand—the links may pull apart. Get a quality leash so that your dog doesn't break it the first time he tries to chase a squirrel. If you take care of them and keep them where your dog can't chew them, the collar and leash will last a long time, so be willing to spend a little more money to get the quality. It's definitely worth it in the long run.

CHAPTER 6

COMMANDS
How to Give Commands Convincingly

Mike taught his white shepherd mix, Ruby, to bow. Every time she stretched, Mike would say, "Take a bow." In time, this became a command, and she would stretch out her front legs and wag her tail above her whenever told to "take a bow." When Mike tried to teach her to pick things up, he used the common command, "take it." She bowed beautifully every time.

WHAT IS A COMMAND?

A command is any word or group of words you choose to tell your dog to complete a specific action. The dictionary defines command as "to direct with authority." Therefore, a command is not a request; it's not "if you feel like doing this, that would be great." A command is: "I'm telling you that this is what you must do now and I expect you to do it."

Your dog doesn't understand English (or Spanish or French or Latin). He will learn to understand many words in your language if you use them consistently. You will discover that you have already taught your dog many words and phrases unintentionally, simply through positive repetition—"ride in the car," "want a cookie," "suppertime." You must now deliberately teach him the commands you want him to learn. If you follow our methods, these commands will also be learned through positive repetition, but there won't be anything accidental in your dog learning them. You'll pick out specific words to convey specific meanings, you'll be consistent in their use, and your dog will come to understand what they mean. For instance, "down" will always mean lie down. It won't sometimes mean "get off the couch" or "don't jump on Aunt Millie."

For any action, you can choose any word in any language. Don't get too complicated or you'll forget the word you're using, and don't use a word that sounds too similar to any other command words or your dog may become confused. Think about what you want your dog to do, think about a word or two that you'll remember easily, then stick with it. In each chapter we'll use the commonly used commands—"sit," "down," "heel,"—but there's no reason why you must use those words.

TONE OF VOICE

Is there a proper way to give a command? The answer is yes. But when someone isn't able to speak or control his voice, he cannot give a command in the traditional way. So the answer is no. Although this book is helpful for everyone who wants to train their dogs, it is written for people with disabilities. Therefore, many variations must be found on traditional training methods in order for a person with a disability to communicate with his or her dog.

DIFFERENT TONES

If you have a full range of voice tones, you'll want to use them in training your dog. This will help convey what you mean. A high, happy voice indicates pleasure. A firm, crisp tone conveys a command. A deep growl communicates disapproval.

Let's look at this from the dog's point of view. When puppies are born, they can't see or hear. One of the first things they begin to hear is the sound of their littermates. They instinctively associate that high-pitched sound with happiness, comfort, and play. Soon they hear their mother's voice, which is deep, firm, but quiet. The puppies associate this voice with authority and guidance.

When you praise your dog in a high, happy voice, he will instinctively become happy. He will recognize the tone of voice long before he knows the words.

When you give a command in a firm, quiet voice, your dog instinctively knows he's around an authority figure. And as soon as you teach him what the command word means, he will obey. When you scold your dog in a deep tone, he will know he has done something to displease you, and if you are consistent in the correction, he'll stop doing it just because you are displeased.

So use as much variation in the inflection in your voice as you are able. Practice different tones in front of your dog. Use nonsense words and watch his reaction. He won't have any idea what you're talking about, but he will recognize communication by your tone. His tail will wag with the high, happy sounds. He will wait expectantly with the authoritative tone. He will lower his tail and head at the deep sounds. You're learning to communicate with your dog using a language he instinctively understands. The better you can use different tones, the easier this communication will be. Remember that the "command" tone is firm and decisive, but quiet.

HOW TO GIVE A COMMAND

One thing you learn quite quickly living with dogs is that they hear very well. Your command doesn't have to be loud. In fact, you want to use as soft a voice as you can. But "soft" doesn't mean sweet or indecisive or hesitant. It just means hushed. You want your command voice to convey authority and control just like your dog's mother was able to convey. So you issue the command in a crisp, firm, strong tone of voice with just enough volume for your dog to hear. Your dog learns to pay close attention to you when you use a quiet voice.

Generally there are four parts to a command: name, command, praise, and release.

Say your dog's name to get his attention and let him know something else is coming.

Issue your one or two word command in a crisp tone, neither too soft nor too loud.

Praise your dog as soon as he completes the action—praise is issued in a high, happy tone of voice, and is followed by a food reward.

Then release him with a word or phrase, like "at ease," "break," or "all done." The release is also given in an upbeat tone. It means that your dog is no longer under the previous command. You always try to get the release word in before your dog "breaks," i.e. moves out of the commanded position. The word "okay" has traditionally been used as a release word, but we don't recommend it. You are very apt to use "okay" frequently in everyday language, and that might be confusing. Remember to praise and give the food reward before the release.

IF YOU HAVE SPEECH DIFFICULTIES

If you cannot form words, you can still train a dog. Even if you cannot make sounds, you can still train a dog.

If you have some speech, your dog will learn to recognize each sound as a distinct command. It doesn't matter if humans can't understand what you just said; your dog will know. And you can change your tone to convey all kinds of messages to your dog.

If you can make sounds, but not words, your dog will learn to understand the subtle differences in the sounds. Try to use the same sound for the same action, and your dog will soon obey. Most important is the change in tone so that he will know when you're pleased with him.

Even if you can't make sounds, you can still communicate with your dog. A smile or a frown, and the body language that

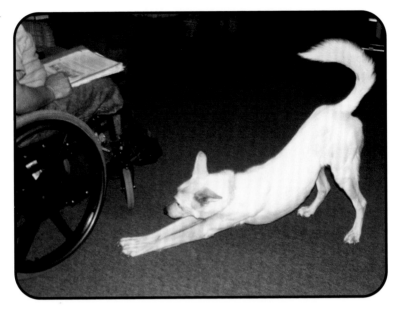

"Take a bow" and "take it" sound so similar that a dog may become
confused. Be careful what command words you choose.
Ruby (white shepherd mix)

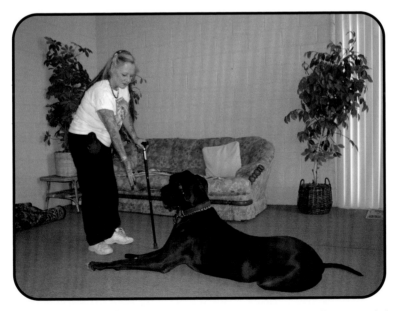

Your commands can all be done with signals, in place of or in addition to verbal
commands. This hand signal for "stay" reminds the dog of the command. Deb
Bettis (bilateral spondylitis of the L5 vertebrae) and Zapata (great Dane)

accompanies them, speak volumes. Dogs can be taught every exercise simply with signals.

SIGNALS

When you say signals to someone in dog obedience, they immediately think of hand signals. But it is not necessary to use your hands to signal your dog. He knows every movement your body makes, knows it better than you do. He watches and understands body language faster and more easily than spoken language. (Be sure to read the section in the "Behavior" chapter on body language (page 29)—it will give you insight into the ways your dog communicates). It's not difficult to teach a dog using signals. You just have to be as consistent as possible, and your dog has to learn to pay close attention to you.

The signals you use for each exercise can be anything that works for you. When you teach the sit as instructed in this book, you are holding a piece of food over your dog's head. That's a signal. When your dog has learned what you want, he will obey the signal with or without food in your hand. When you teach down according to this book, your hand signal is bringing the food to the floor. Again, that becomes the command even if you are unable to utter a word. If you're in a power chair, the click of your motor is a signal to your dog to move. No words are necessary.

If you have good hand and arm movement you can use fairly broad signals at first, exaggerating each movement so your dog can easily see it. As he learns the command you can make the movements smaller so he will learn to pay even closer attention. Remember to be consistent—one signal for each command. Even if you have a lot of involuntary movement, you can still approximate the same movement every time for each command. Despite extra motion, your dog will come to recognize the signal.

If you have trouble moving your hands and arms, you can use your legs and feet as signals. Stewart, in a wheelchair, separated his legs as he gave the "come" command. This was an extra signal that he could use if he was unable to get the sound out. His dogs knew it meant "come." You may only be able to use your eyes and face. You can work out a system where rolling your eyes up means "sit," rolling your eyes down means "down," and dropping your head means "stay." This would have to be coupled at first with teaching your dog what "sit" and "down" and "stay" mean, and it would probably take longer for your dog to recognize such subtle signals, but he can learn.

You will have to devise the signals that work for you. It doesn't matter what signal you choose. If you use the same signal as consistently as you can to mean the same command every time, your dog will learn it.

Throughout this book, when we say "tell your dog to sit," for instance, it means use words if you can, sounds if you can't make words, and signals if you can't make sounds. It means do whatever you have to do to convey the idea to your dog. And be as consistent as you can to use the same word/sound/signal to mean the same thing every time.

CHAPTER 7

ATTENTION
Teach Your Dog to Look at You, Bond with You, Obey You

Mike was trying to train Etta Jane, a strong-willed cattle dog mix. She had sharp herding tendencies, a very alert nature, and a potential to protect. Mike had to find a way to redirect her energy. He began teaching "attention" using food and praise, saying her name, an attention command, and giving her a treat every time she looked at him. She attacked this exercise with the same intensity she put into everything. Within a few days, Mike found her staring at him constantly, with such single-minded concentration that it began to make him self-conscious. A trained counselor, he considered therapy for both of them.

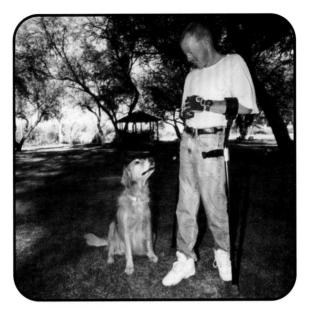

When you have your dog's undivided attention
all training is easier and more fun.
Blake Gigli (spinal cord injury T 12) and
Savannah (golden retriever)

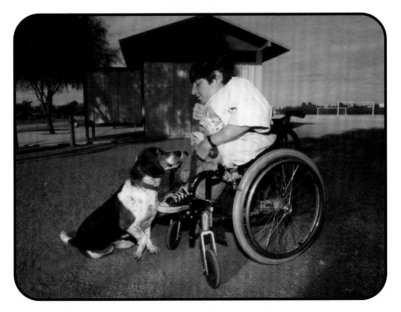

Amazingly, even a beagle can be taught to pay attention to his owner.
Mary Jane Cera (osteogenesis imperfecta) and Barney (beagle mix)

ATTENTION, PLEASE

You now have a much better understanding of your dog, and you're probably anxious to begin training him. Before you can teach your dog anything, however, you must get him to look at you so that he is ready to receive the command. It's vital for anyone who wants to teach in a positive manner. You need to devise a way to get your dog to look at you dependably. You need your dog's undivided attention.

The first exercise you will teach your dog is called "attention," and it can be any word, or sound, or movement that gets his attention. First, you will give a command, such as "Toby, watch me," or "Daisy, look." Then find a way to make him want to look at you. You could click your tongue or make "kissing" sounds. You could make a high-pitched noise and smile at the same time. You could whistle. You could pat your leg. You could click a clicker or rattle your keys. As soon as your dog looks at you, you praise, verbally, if possible, or with a smile or a pat, and give a food treat.

Please understand that this is an exercise to be learned and practiced, just like "sit" and "down" and "come." You must work on this two or three times a day, every day, until your dog is consistently looking at you.

TEACHING ATTENTION

Begin in a quiet place with no distractions. Have a lot of small food treats handy—and we do mean a lot. Refer to the "Food" chapter to help you decide what treat to use and how to dispense it. Remember that timing is important, but if you're slow or if someone has to help you give the food, your dog will still learn that a treat follows this action. Most important, remember that appropriate praise always comes first, as quickly as you can give it.

You want to teach your dog that when you say a word, such as "look" or "watch me," it means that you want your dog to look up into your face. When he learns to do that readily, you'll have his total attention, and he will be ready to receive your next command.

Say your dog's name, followed by the attention command. If possible, show him a treat in your hand and move it up in front of your face. This will usually cause him to follow the treat and look at your face. As soon as he looks at you, praise enthusiastically and give him the treat. Pop the treat in his mouth as quickly as you are able. Practice this for a minute or two. That doesn't mean you want your dog to look at you for two minutes! You're only asking him to look at you for a second each time. Keep repeating the command, moving the treat to your face and/or making noises to get him to look. Praise and reward every time he looks at you.

You must be very alert to your dog during this exercise. If he looks at you on his own, you must praise and reward him. It sounds easy to praise your dog each time, but it takes a lot of concentration on your part. If your dog looks at you several times and receives no reward, he will respond more slowly next time. He has to be taught that this is the action you want, and in order for him to learn that, you must reward him appropriately.

If you're unable to bring your hands up to your face, you'll have to use your voice to make sounds that make him look at you. Or you can have a friend hold the food close to your face. If you have to use a friend, you must train that person to do his or her part correctly. Your friend should stand very close to you with a handful of treats. You give the attention command, and as soon as your dog looks at you, you give appropriate praise. Then your friend places a treat on your lap, or, if necessary, gives your dog the treat. It's important for your friend to wait until you have praised before giving the treat. Your dog will know that your friend has the food, but he will also quickly learn that he only gets the treat when he has looked at you. This system can work well. You're still doing all the training; you're just using your friend as a training tool.

Do whatever it takes to get your dog to look into your face, and don't give him the reward until he does. He will quickly learn what brings the praise and food treat, and he will begin to look at you automatically, hoping to elicit the response. That's why you must pay as close attention to him as you're asking him to pay to you. Remember to praise each time he looks at you.

If you're unable to do anything to arouse your dog's attention, just use the times when he looks at you on his own. As soon as he looks, say "good look," and give him a food reward. Keep paying close attention to him so you don't miss any times he looks at you.

JACKPOT

Jackpot is a concept taken from the slot machines at casinos all around the world. The thrill is when the machine pays off with a big reward. Bells ring, lights flash, and everyone is aware that something special has happened. In dog training, you can use this concept to excite your dog. No bells or lights, but a handful, or jackpot, of treats.

As you're working on the attention command, and all future commands, there will be times when your dog does the exercise under difficult circumstances. You give your attention command just as the cat comes in the room. If your dog looks at you instead of the cat, he deserves a jackpot of treats. This will excite him and make him want to look at you even more readily next time. When you've taught your dog the sit command and a lady approaches in a fancy dress, you see that your dog with muddy paws is about to jump up on her. You say "sit," in your most commanding voice, and your dog sits. You're so pleased (and amazed) that you give your dog all the treats in your hand. That's a jackpot. Your dog obeyed your command instantly and under difficult circumstances (he really wanted to greet the lady). So his reward is commensurate with the accomplishment.

You can use jackpotting in all areas of training. If your dog finds any exercise difficult, you can jackpot each advance. This will make him more inclined to repeat the exercise correctly. It makes for a happier, more positive atmosphere for learning.

STAGE TWO

When your dog is looking at you quickly and consistently whenever you give your attention command, move on to stage two. Now your dog will begin to learn how to learn; he will figure out on his own, without prompting from you, what brings reward.

Set up to do the exercise just as you've been doing—food ready, in a quiet setting. Don't say anything to your dog. He will recognize the circumstances and will probably look at you quite readily. Praise—"good look"—and reward with a treat, then remain quiet. As soon as he looks at you again, praise enthusiastically and reward.

If he doesn't look at you after about thirty seconds, give your attention signal and praise when he looks. Any time he looks at you without the attention signal, give very enthusiastic praise and several treats. This jackpot effect will make him more inclined to look at you readily.

Remember that you must reward with praise and food every time he looks at you. Keep treats handy around the house so that you can reward him in other places and other times. You're asking your dog to understand that you want him to want to look at you. He doesn't have to wait for an invitation; he's going to get rewarded when he remembers to do it on his own. This also makes you much more aware of your dog since you have to be watching for him to watch you.

PERFECTING ATTENTION

When your dog readily looks at you, you can work with distractions. Have a friend stand a few feet away and clap his hands to entice your dog. You give your attention command. Your dog should be so well-conditioned to praise and treats that he turns to you without hesitation. If he's more interested in your friend, you haven't worked long enough or consistently enough. Go back to basics.

If he looks at you and ignores your friend, praise and give him a jackpot of treats. Practice this several times, keeping yourself more enthusiastic and more interesting than your friend. This will help get your dog's attention back on you whenever he is distracted by anything.

The more you practice this, the better you will bond as a team. The more you notice your dog looking at you and reward him for it, the more aware you are of each other. Remember that your dog is going to school, and you're the teacher. The student will learn much faster if he is paying attention to the teacher. Think of this as an ongoing exercise. Don't stop practicing just because your dog has learned to look at you. It's a connection that needs to be reinforced and rewarded throughout your dog's lifetime.

CHAPTER 8

SIT
Teach Your Dog to Sit on Command

The great Dane, Forego, was huge. He came into class dragging his frail owner behind him. But Michael loved his dog so much. He was somewhat insulted when the instructor, Mike, hinted that Forego might be out of control. To prove him wrong, Michael brought Forego over to Mike, who is in a wheelchair. Michael commanded, "Forego, sit," in a nice authoritative voice. Forego backed up and sat perfectly—in Mike's lap!

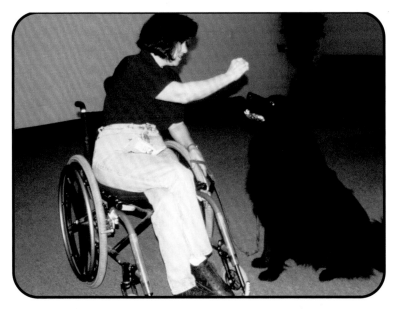

The easiest way to teach your dog to sit is to use food held just over his head. Linda Ferguson (spinal cord injury T 12) and Hootie (chow/Newfoundland)

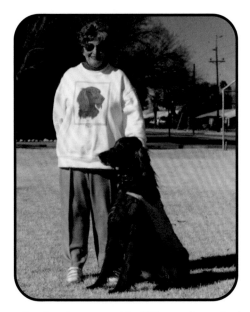

You must practice the sit command in different places. It gives your dog more confidence. Claire Weeks (arthritis) and Tray (Irish setter)

WHAT IS A SIT?

Sit is the position when the dog's rump is resting on a surface. It may be that the dog sits with his hips shifted to one side, or he may sit perfectly square. That is not as important as the fact that he is settled in a sit position.

A dog has to learn what the word means before it becomes a command. Just because you know what sit means, don't assume that your dog does. He must be taught. But understand that you're not teaching your dog to sit; he knows how to sit. You're teaching him to do it when you tell him to. You're teaching him what the word "sit" means.

TEACHING THE SIT

The easiest, most positive way to teach sit is with food. Most dogs like to work for treats and are very responsive, but some go completely out of control over food. If you have a dog who simply gets crazy whenever food is around, you must bring this under control before you can begin to teach him anything. Please refer to the "Food" chapter (page 18) for tips on working with this situation, and get it under control before you try to teach any exercise.

To teach sit, hold a piece of food above your dog's head just out of reach. Don't hold it too high or your dog will jump up for it. Move it slightly back over his head. As he watches the food overhead, he will usually sink into the sit position. It might take a minute or two for this to happen, so be patient. Keep holding the food just above his head. As soon as his rump hits the floor, say, "sit, good sit," and give him the food treat. Remember that if you have difficulty speaking, you must find a sound or signal to mean "sit" and use it consistently.

Your dog doesn't have to stay seated for more than a second. The command comes as he sits, not before. He doesn't know what the word means. Be sure to give appropriate praise.

If you are unable to hold a piece of food above your dog, you might get someone to hold it for you, or you might devise a method of holding food in a container. See the chapter on "Food" for some ideas, and don't hesitate to be inventive.

If your dog tends to move around following the food instead of sitting, get him against a wall or in a corner. Don't back him into a corner if he seems threatened by this, but if you talk to him in a high, happy voice and show him the food, you can usually prevent him from being nervous in this situation. Hold the food patiently just above his head and keep talking to him. If he wants the food and has nowhere to go, he will usually sink into a sit. Give the command and praise as he sits, followed immediately by the food treat. Then let him out of the corner, and try again later. It will usually only take a time or two before a clever dog learns that the act of sitting gets him the treat.

As part of teaching your dog what the word sit means, you may actually use feeding time as a training tool. If you are able, hold up your dog's bowl just over his head and command "sit" as he sits. As soon as he sits, give appropriate praise and place the food bowl in front of him. Then use a word as he begins eating, like "supper" or "okay, eat" or something else that you will use consistently. Again, he won't have any idea what it means, but you will soon have control of his feeding.

Be consistent in working on the sit. Always have a food treat in the early stages of training, until you are absolutely sure your dog knows the command. Always give the command word. And always give appropriate praise.

PRAISE

The verbal praise must be given before the food. Don't think the food is enough. Your dog must always have appropriate praise from you. There will be situations where you won't have food, but you can always praise your dog. And remember that "appropriate" means appropriate for you and your dog. Remember to use the command as part of the praise—say "good sit" rather than just "good dog." It will reinforce the command. If you cannot speak, your praise should be a sound, a gesture, or a movement that conveys pleasure. Use the same signal to mean praise every time.

RELEASE

As soon as you have praised your dog appropriately and given him the food treat, use a release word as discussed in the "Command" chapter (page 62). Be consistent in the word you choose—like "break" or "release" or "at ease." Your dog will have no idea what that means now, but he will come to learn that it means he no longer has to continue with the previous command. Use an excited high-pitched tone for the release word. You must give your release word before your dog moves from the commanded position. You want him to move only on your command, not because he chooses to.

PERFECTING THE SIT

After a few repetitions, your dog will probably sit automatically as soon as you pull out a food treat. This doesn't mean he's learned the sit command; it just means he's smart enough to know one sure way to get a treat. Get him on his feet. Back away from him—he will follow you for the food. As soon as he's following you, give him the sit command, then as soon as he sits, praise him. Wait several seconds before you give him the food treat. He must stay seated during this period. If he gets up, tell him sit again, and praise when he sits, but hold the food. After he has sat for several seconds, give appropriate praise and the food treat; then release him.

Work on this step for a week before you move on, even if your dog responds quickly. If he doesn't sit at all, go back to the first step—holding the food over his head. Be sure you give the sit command firmly as he sits, so he will associate the word with the action.

Next, vary the length of time between his response to the command and his getting the food reward (remember always to verbally praise as soon as he responds). This is not a stay. You are not leaving your dog. You are just expecting him to remain seated until you are ready to reward him with the food. You must remember to give him the release command. As soon as you verbally praise him and give him the treat, say your release word in a happy voice so that he knows the exercise is over. It's okay if he stays sitting, but it's also okay if he gets up.

Work on these varying lengths of time until you are certain that your dog really knows what sit means and that he sits as soon as he hears you say the word.

To test this, don't take out a piece of food, and make sure your dog knows you don't have one in your hand. Give the command "sit" and watch his response. If you've been consistent in your commands and your praise, and if you've worked on it long enough, your dog should respond quickly to the command. Give immediate appropriate praise, and pull out a food treat. If he doesn't sit promptly, go back to the beginning and build up slowly.

When your dog is responding promptly to the sit command, you can begin to taper off the food reward. Give him a treat every other time. Always give appropriate praise whether you give food or not. Then you can give food for every third or fourth sit, followed by giving it at random. You should never eliminate the food reward altogether. Your dog should always have hope that he might get a food treat.

Keep practicing sit as you begin to teach other commands. Even when you're working on advanced exercises, you want to practice these basic commands often. Once he understands and obeys the sit command every time, you can use it whenever you're in strange or difficult circumstances. Sit is comfortable and familiar, and it will put you in control of the situation.

CHAPTER 9

DOWN
Teach Your Dog to Lie Down on Command

Stewart and his border collie, Annie, were coming out of a restaurant. The ramp was quite steep—Stewart needed his friend Kathy to hold back on his power chair as he descended. It was also so narrow that Annie couldn't walk beside him. The only solution was to send Annie ahead while Stewart and Kathy brought the chair down slowly and safely. Stewart told Annie "away," and she obediently went ahead. When she got beyond the bottom of the ramp, probably twenty feet away, Stewart commanded, "Down!" which Annie obeyed instantly. Stewart and Kathy could then concentrate on bringing the chair down cautiously, knowing that Annie would remain patiently in the down position until Stewart could get to her and release her.

WHAT DOES DOWN MEAN?

Down is when your dog is in a lying-down position all the way on the ground. It doesn't matter if he is lying on his back, side, or stomach. It just matters that he is, in fact, down.

In the beginning, you simply teach your dog what the word down means; you're not expecting him to stay down for any length of time.

This may be the hardest exercise for your dog to learn. It is the most submissive position a dog can be in, and your dog may be reluctant to assume the position. Don't get into a power struggle with him; just follow these methods to teach him what the word means.

TEACHING THE DOWN

There are several methods for teaching the down. Decide which will work best for you and your dog. Always get yourself totally prepared for the exercise before you ever give the command. This means your dog should be on leash and the food treats are within easy reach ready to be dispensed.

You may want to fasten the leash to something secure or sit on it so you don't have to worry about it. This way you can be sure your dog won't get the food before he's done the exercise, and he can't leave the area.

Method 1

If you can reach all the way to the floor, this is the easiest method. With a piece of food in your hand, put your hand just in front of your dog's nose and move your hand slowly outward and downward. His head will automatically come forward and down, following your hand. It's very important, therefore, to move your hand slowly and not abruptly jerk it to the floor.

As your dog's head is moving down, give the command "down" and begin to praise—using the words "good down" if you are able. Be patient and move your hand slowly. Put your other hand gently on his shoulders to encourage him to go down. Keep the food just out of his reach. Be prepared for your dog to put his rear end up in the air as his head is coming down. Many dogs do this. Just

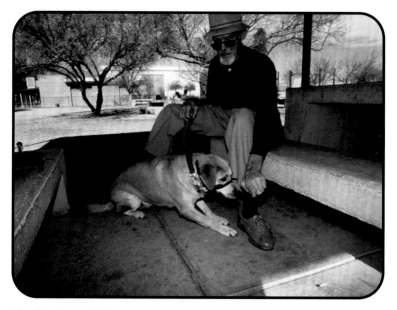

Food is a great help when teaching the down exercise. Your dog will follow your hand to the ground and lie down without a struggle. Jack Stumpenhorst (polio) and Missy (lab mix)

patiently hold the food at ground level and don't let him have it until both ends are down.

As soon as he lies down, and we mean the second his belly hits the floor, give appropriate praise followed immediately by the treat. Give the treat from your hand, if possible, not from the floor. You want your dog to know it comes from you, and you don't want him to get in the habit of eating things off the floor. If the only way you can give a treat is from the floor, then do that, but that should be a last resort. Try other methods of dispensing food first.

Method 2

Depending on your disability it may be difficult or impossible for you to reach the floor. The next best thing is to get your dog up to your height. Before you can teach the down, you may need to teach him to get up on a piece of furniture. Give a command like "up" or "jump," hold a food treat over the sofa and pat the surface. Praise if your dog puts his front paws up and keep encouraging him. When he hops up, give appropriate praise and the food treat.

Having your dog at this height makes it easier for you to reach him, and it works on his natural instinct not to fall. Dogs explore edges carefully and will not fall off something on purpose, so you need to be very careful not to let your dog, especially a small dog, fall off the sofa or bed, or he'll associate the exercise with that bad experience.

Hold the food in front of your dog's nose, and move your hand slowly away and down. This way his head will automatically come forward and down, following your hand. It's very important, therefore, to move your hand slowly, not abruptly jerk it down. If you move it too fast, he will probably jump off the sofa to try and get the food. Hold the treat just below the edge of the sofa. Put your other hand gently on his shoulders to encourage him to go down and also to keep him on the sofa. As he lowers his head, give the command "down," and begin to praise—using the words "good down" if you are able. Be patient and move your hand slowly. Keep the food just out of his reach.

As soon as your dog lies down on the sofa, the instant his belly is down, give appropriate praise and the food. Don't let the food drop to the floor or he will jump down after it. You want him to know the food comes from you and is a reward for lying down, not jumping off the sofa. In this case, you must devise some means of giving him the treat on the sofa.

PRAISE

Always remember that the praise must be given before the food. Don't think the food is enough. Your dog must always hear appropriate praise from you. There will be situations when you don't have food, but you can always praise your dog.

RELEASE

Remember to use your release word as soon as you have praised your dog appropriately and given him the food treat. At first, release him immediately. As you practice this exercise, you can begin to wait several seconds before releasing him. You must give your release word before your dog moves from the commanded position. You want him to move only on your command, not because he chooses to.

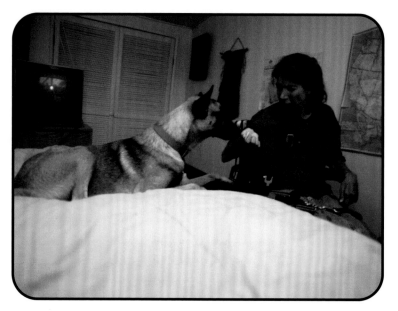

Getting your dog up on a bed or sofa may be an easier way for you to teach the down. Dianne Kalal (spinal cord injury C 5-6) and Radar(Belgian malinois)

PERFECTING THE DOWN

You will need to practice the down exercise faithfully. Do two or three downs in succession and then play with your dog or practice something else. Then do two or three more. After a week or two of diligent practice, you must begin a transition.

If you used method 1, you now need to begin to bend less and less. Your dog must learn to obey the down command without you having to bend all the way to the floor. You will teach this by alternating how far you bend.

If you've been standing beside your dog, and bending way over, you might try working from a chair with your dog sitting beside you. Give the down command firmly and move your hand three-fourths of the way to the floor. As soon as your dog obeys the command, give appropriate praise and move your hand down to give him the food reward. Don't let him sit up to take the food. He must get the treat while still in the down position. Then practice a down where you put your hand all the way to the floor as you give the command.

Practice several downs at the three-quarter level; then try moving your hand only halfway to the floor. If your dog stops at the level of your hand, you must work longer to teach him what the word down means. But if he obeys the verbal command, he must hear immediate appropriate praise and get a food reward. Your goal is to be able to say "down," point to the floor, and have your dog go right down.

If you cannot speak and you are teaching down exclusively with signals, you might want to slowly diminish your signal. This will be easier on you, and will also result in your dog paying closer attention to you.

If you used method 2, the transition is usually easier. Work on the sofa for at least a week, faithfully giving the down command, praise, and reward. Then sit in a chair and try giving the command with your dog sitting beside you. You may lower your hand, with food in it, toward the floor. If your dog has learned the word, he should go into the down position readily. Give appropriate praise and the food treat. Concentrate on not bending, but just pointing to the floor.

Continue to practice sit and down several times each day, but don't always do them one after the other. If you always have down follow every sit, your dog may begin to anticipate and simply lie down when you tell him to sit. You want him to learn each command word separately.

When your dog is readily going into position in response to your verbal command, and holding the position for a few seconds until you release him, you are ready to begin teaching "stay."

CHAPTER 10

STAY

Teach Your Dog to Remain in the Sit or Down Position until Released

Stewart's lab, Beverly, was a well-trained obedience dog, easily scoring well at dog shows. One day while practicing sit stays, Bev uncharacteristically got up and moved. Stewart went quickly to her and put her back in the place he had left her. He wheeled away with a firm "stay" command. He was astonished when she again got up and moved. Stewart knew that the only way to correct such a bad habit was to put her right back in place and insist that she obey the command. Some trainers blindly follow that rule, but Stewart began to wonder why his normally obedient dog was disobeying such a basic command. Instead of correcting, Stewart evaluated the situation and found that he had made her sit on top of an anthill. She had obeyed and tolerated the discomfort for as long as she could each time; then she had felt the need to move. Stewart put her on a sit stay a few feet away, and she sat perfectly for three minutes.

WHAT IS STAY?

Stay means that your dog maintains both his position and place until you give him another command or release him. In other words, if your dog is sitting and you tell him to stay, he must remain in the sit position in that exact spot. This exercise cannot be attempted until your dog is obeying sit and down promptly with one verbal command, and not popping back up immediately. You must be certain he understands the sit and down commands before he can be expected to learn the stay.

To test this, command your dog to sit. When he does, praise quietly and remain as still as possible beside him while you count to yourself to ten. If your dog moves from the sit, you need to practice longer on just the sit. If he remains seated, give appropriate praise and release him. Do the same thing with the down command. He should be calm and relaxed in both positions before you try to teach stay.

Don't rush into this exercise, or you'll find it very difficult for your dog to learn. If your dog isn't ready for stay, move on to other exercises while continuing to practice sit and down. Come back to stay in a couple of weeks when your dog is more settled.

UNDERSTANDING STAY

It's important for you to really understand the stay before you can be expected to teach it to your dog. You need to have a picture in your mind of what you expect him to do. At first, he will have no idea what you want, and if you're confused about what you're asking, imagine how confused he must be.

The stay must progress very slowly. That means you will not physically leave your dog right away. It's important that you don't move too far from him while he's learning an exercise. This is what too often happens: You say "stay" and move away. Your dog gets up and follows you because he has no idea what stay means. You fumble with the leash, shout "no," turn around, position him again, shout "stay," and move away again. Now your dog is really confused. The only thing he can think to do is go with you and hope that will please you. When it doesn't and you get angrier, your dog will become more and more unsure of himself.

Remember that you want to build up positives in your dog and set him up to succeed, not to fail. You want to build his confidence so that when you do step away from him, he will have the poise to remain where he is. Every dog is different, every trainer is different, every exercise is different. We don't know how long it will take you to teach this exercise, but although you can read through the whole chapter in a few minutes, expect to spend days on each step.

The difficulty in teaching stay is that it's a different concept from other training exercises. With sit and down, you lure your dog into moving into a specific position. He learns to do something when he hears "sit," and he gets rewarded when he does. With stay, he has to learn not to do something, in fact, not to do anything. It's a harder concept to teach. So just take it slow and steady and err on the side of too much practice on each step rather than too little.

Remember in dog training, "slow is fast."

TEACHING THE STAY

There are different methods to use depending on your disability, but everyone should begin the same way. Command your dog to sit. Give appropriate praise. (Always praise your dog for each position, even though another command will follow). Command your dog "stay."

If you have the physical ability, you may use your hand as a stay signal. With your hand flat, or as flat as you can get it (if your fingers are curled, your dog may think you have food), place your hand, palm first, in front of your dog's nose. It's just an extra signal that you can use as you say "stay." It may act as a barrier in front of your dog. It's not mandatory; you must decide if it's a help or a hindrance.

Do not move. Stay as quietly as possible beside your dog and count to yourself to three. Quietly praise or signal "good stay." Then release your dog. It's generally easier not to use food on the stay, because it can be quite distracting to your dog. But if you do use food, be sure to give the food reward while your dog is staying, before you release him. You want him to know that the reward is for the stay, not for the release.

Move around with your dog, and then repeat the exercise. This time, count to five. Most important, do not move during the stay. If your dog moves before the count of five, go back and practice several times at the count of three until he's reliable.

At this point, your dog has no concept of what he did right, but as you consistently practice, he will begin to get the idea. If he starts to get up or lie down, you are right there to correct him by repeating the sit command firmly and then repeating the stay command. In fact, you can watch him and firmly repeat "stay" if you even think he's going to move. Remember that firm doesn't mean loud.

By being right beside him, you are able to anticipate his moves and you're close enough to effectively stop him from breaking. This is the idea of teaching your dog the exercise so thoroughly that he will not make a mistake. Use firm but quiet commands or signals with the stay exercise conveying your confidence that he will do it correctly. Praise should also be quiet, not boisterous.

Now, down your dog. Praise for the down. Command "stay" and use your hand signal. Do not move. Count to yourself to three, praise "good stay," and release. Move around with your dog, and then repeat. This time count to five. If your dog moves before the count of five, go back and practice several times at the count of three until he's reliable.

If your dog does the sit very well, but won't stay down, you can teach stay just from the sit position. Keep working on down until he becomes reliable, and then you can work on the down stay. Otherwise, practice stay alternating sit and down positions. Build up the time your dog remains in the stay. Build up slowly until he will stay reliably for one minute. You're still right next to your dog.

Before you begin to leave your dog, you need to develop the positive attitude that he will do what you tell him. Believe that he is going to stay and he will. That's why you practice so long on the stay with him right beside you. Both of you gain confidence and poise.

How you teach the stay will depend on your circumstances. We have broken the exercise into four sections: ambulatory, ambulatory with devices, manual wheelchair, and power chair. Turn to the one that is most appropriate for your situation, and read that section. It will give you the steps to teach your dog to stay and will address specific difficulties and solutions for each circumstance.

LEAVING YOUR DOG
Ambulatory

Command your dog to sit. Give appropriate praise. Command "stay," and take a small step away from your dog to the side. Immediately step back beside him, quietly praise, then release. Walk around with him, and then repeat the sequence.

If your dog breaks, you have not spent enough time working on stay beside him. Don't rush. It's much more difficult to go back and start over than to do it right the first time.

Gradually increase the time that you spend one step away from your dog until he is staying for a full minute.

Next, command your dog to sit. Then command "stay." Take the small step to the side, then step in front of your dog and turn to face him. You should just pivot in front of him so you're right there ready to make a correction if he starts to break. Quietly praise—"good stay"—then pivot back beside him. Again, quietly praise and then release him.

He should not break the stay when you return to his side or when he hears the praise. He should not move until he hears the release word. If he breaks before that, you must get him back in position, repeat the stay command, and leave him, but not as far or for as long.

When your dog is thoroughly reliable on this step, give him the stay command and/or signal, and walk straight ahead four feet, turn and face him. Be sure that you don't pull the leash tight as you walk away.

Don't hesitate to repeat the stay command and/or signal when you face him. (If you've been able to use the hand signal with the stay command, this is when it becomes most helpful. You can simply point your hand, palm first, at your dog as the reminder to stay.) Count to yourself to ten and return beside him. Again, don't hesitate to repeat the stay as you return to him. Quietly praise and release.

At each of these stages, practice sometimes in sit and sometimes in down so your dog will learn to stay in any position.

Now it's just a matter of building up time. A dog can easily stay in a sit for several minutes and a down for half an hour or more. Practice stay in different locations and for varying lengths of time, but remember to be aware of circumstances. Don't expect your dog to sit stay on a slippery floor or on top of an anthill. Don't put him in a down stay in a busy doorway. You always want to set yourself up to succeed. Think of each new location as a brand new exercise and proceed through the steps of the stay in each place.

LEAVING YOUR DOG
Ambulatory with Devices

If you use canes, crutches, a walker, or any other device to help your mobility, you will need to approach the stay a little more cautiously than if you walk unaided. Even if you use a device only part of the time, be sure to practice each exercise using the device so your dog gets used to it. Your dog may have a solid sit stay, but the first time you drop your crutch on him while he's staying, you may have to start all over again.

If you use a cane or crutches most or all of the time, chances are they have already fallen on or near your dog at least once. Any time your crutch falls on him, you need to express your sympathy in a high-pitched, happy voice. If you coddle your dog, you'll just reinforce his apprehension around the crutches.

If he has become fearful of your crutches, you may have to build up his confidence so that he will stay even when you start moving your crutch. (Crutch is used from here on to convey any walking aid). Remember also that your dog is used to going with you when you move your crutches.

When he is staying beside you for one minute, practice dropping your crutch beside you but away from him. Begin this on a carpeted surface so the crutch won't clatter or bounce toward your dog. You may want to sit in a chair beside him to practice this so you won't lose your balance. Say "stay" as you drop the crutch, and be prepared to repeat the command and correct him. If he remains sitting, praise profusely, then release. If he gets up, but sits back down on command, give appropriate praise, then release. Next, practice two or three sit stays without dropping a crutch. Now, down your dog. Say "stay" as you drop the crutch, and be prepared

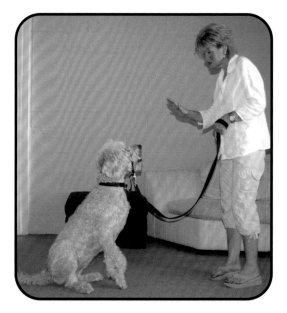

If your dog starts to move, be quick to remind him
to "sit" and "stay." Diane Manchester
(multiple sclerosis) and Mojo (labradoodle).

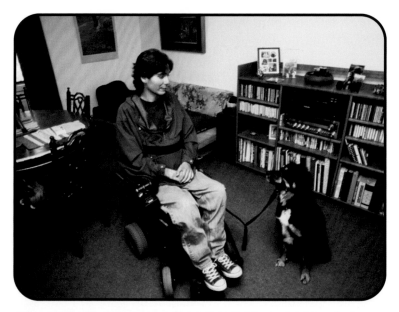

When you're able to leave your dog on the sit stay, go about four feet away
and turn at a 45 degree angle. Chris Wenner (spinal cord injury C 5-6)
and Koa (Australian shepherd)

to repeat the command and correct him. Dogs consider down a vulnerable position, so he's very apt to move when you drop the crutch. Be patient. Always make sure that you drop it well away from him.

During some stays, practice moving the crutch in front of and beside your dog. Don't move yourself, just the crutch. He must learn to be confident around the crutches and also learn not to move once he has heard the stay command. This will take time since he has probably keyed in to the movement of the crutches. Say "stay" firmly (not loudly) each time you move or drop the crutch. And always give appropriate praise.

When your dog ignores the crutches and remains in the stay reliably, command "stay," and take one very small step away from your dog to the side. Immediately step back beside him, quietly praise, then release. Walk around with him, and then repeat the sequence.

If your dog breaks, you have not spent enough time working on stay beside him. Don't rush. It's much more difficult to go back and start over than to do it right the first time.

Gradually increase the time that you spend one step away from your dog until he is staying for one minute.

Next, command your dog to sit. Then command "stay." Take the small step to the side, then step in front of your dog and turn to face him. You should just pivot in front of him, as much as your crutches or walker will allow. You want to be right there ready to make a correction if he starts to break. Quietly praise—"good stay"—then pivot back beside him. Again, quietly praise and then release him.

He should not break the stay when you return to his side or when he hears the praise. He should not move until he hears the release word. If he breaks before that, you must get him back in position, repeat the stay command, and leave him, but not as far or for as long.

During these practice sessions, you must be very careful not to drop the crutch on your dog or hit him with the crutches as you leave or return to him. If you do, understand that this may be a big setback. Be sure to use a happy voice when you apologize. Then go back to working on stays beside you until you build his confidence again. Don't rush him if he is shy of your crutches; it will not help in the long run. Make the training sessions positive and happy. Also be sure the leash doesn't become tangled in the crutch and pull on your dog.

When your dog is thoroughly reliable on this step, give him the stay command and/or signal and walk straight ahead four feet, turn and face him. Be sure that you don't pull the leash tight as you walk away.

Don't hesitate to repeat the stay command and/or signal when you face him. (If you've been able to use the hand signal with the stay command, this is when it becomes most helpful. You can simply point your hand, palm first, at your dog as the reminder to stay.) Count to yourself to ten and return beside him. Again, don't hesitate to repeat the stay as you return to him. Quietly praise and release.

At each of these stages, practice sometimes in sit and sometimes in down so your dog will learn to stay in any position.

Now it's just a matter of building up time. A dog can easily stay in a sit for several minutes and a down for half an hour or more. Practice stay in different locations and for varying lengths of time, but remember to be aware of circumstances. Don't expect your dog to sit stay on a slippery floor or on top of an anthill. Don't put him in a down stay in a busy doorway. You always want to set yourself up to succeed. Think of each new location as a brand new exercise and proceed through the steps of the stay in each place.

LEAVING YOUR DOG
Manual Wheelchair

Remember that your dog is used to going beside you when you roll your chair, and he's also used to getting out of the way of your chair. That's why stay is more difficult to teach from a wheelchair. It will take more patience on your part and perhaps more time. Any time you roll over your dog, you need to express your sympathy in a high-pitched, happy voice. If you coddle your dog, it will only reinforce his fear of the wheelchair. Unless he's really hurt, he will snap out of it much faster if you don't give him reason to continue crying. And you'll know if he's really hurt.

Command your dog to sit. Give appropriate praise. Command stay.

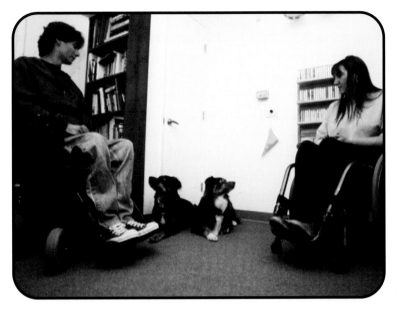

Chris and LeNae trained their dogs together. Note the attention each dog is paying to its owner. Chris Wenner (spinal cord injury C 5-6) and Koa (Australian shepherd) and LeNae Liebetrau (spinal cord injury T 10) and Miki (Australian shepherd)

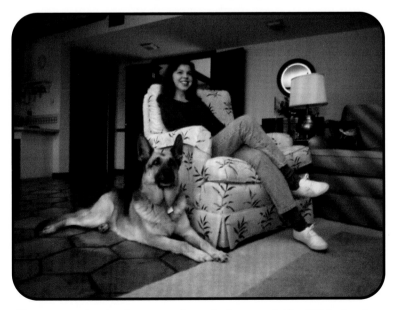

You can practice the down stay when relaxing or watching TV. Just make sure your dog stays down until you release him. Kellie Christenson (juvenile rheumatoid arthritis) and Atlee (German shepherd)

Be sure to check your dog's position before you touch your wheels. If he is too close for you to move, release him from the stay and try again. It's important that there be no contact between your dog and your wheelchair. If there is, you must be understanding if your dog gets out of the way.

When he's positioned so you won't touch him with the chair, command "stay," and move the chair forward just the slightest bit, angling away from your dog. You will barely move. Roll back beside your dog and quietly praise—"good stay"—then release him. Move around with your dog and then repeat the sequence.

If your dog breaks, you have not spent enough time working on stay beside him. Don't rush. It's much more difficult to go back and start over than to do it right the first time.

Gradually increase the time that you spend on this first step until he is staying for a full minute.

Now you will roll about a foot forward, angling away from your dog. Immediately roll back beside him and give quiet praise. Then release him.

He should not break the stay when you return to his side or when he hears the praise. He should not move until he hears the release word. If he breaks before that, you must get him back in position, repeat the stay command, and leave him, but not as far or for as long.

Increase the time that you can stay in this position slowly. If you do it right and don't rush, each step will occur more quickly. Your dog is understanding what you want. Remember to praise, using the words "good stay," while you're away from him.

Now roll about four feet forward and turn your chair at a right angle to him. Be careful that the leash doesn't pull tight as you roll forward.

Don't hesitate to repeat the stay command and/or signal when you face him. (If you've been able to use the hand signal with the stay command, this is when it becomes most helpful. You can simply point your hand, palm first, at your dog as the reminder to stay.) Count to yourself to ten and return beside him. Again, don't hesitate to repeat the stay as you return to him. Quietly praise and release.

If he shifts position to avoid the wheels as you leave him but doesn't move out of the sit, give the command again as a reminder and praise "good stay." If he seems leery of the wheelchair as you return to him, practice by rolling toward him very slowly as you remind him to stay, and praise quietly.

Next, command your dog to stay, go forward at least four feet and turn to face him. Some wheelchairs have footrests that stick out a foot or more from the chair. Be sure that there is no danger of the footrests hitting him when you turn to face him. That's why you turn at a right angle to your dog first. You can gauge the distance. If you have protruding footrests, go farther away before you turn to face him.

The other thing you need to be aware of when leaving your dog is that the leash should never pull tight. This would be an unfair signal to him. He must decide whether to obey the stay command or the tug on the leash. Before you leave him, be sure you have enough slack and be careful that it doesn't get caught in the wheels or the footrests.

At each of these stages, practice sometimes in sit and sometimes in down so your dog will learn to stay in any position.

When he is staying reliably when you turn to face him, begin to build up the time that you leave him in this position. A dog can easily stay in a sit for several minutes and a down for half an hour or more. Practice stay in different locations and for varying lengths of time, but remember to be aware of circumstances. Don't expect your dog to sit stay on a slippery floor or on top of an anthill. Don't put him in a down stay in a busy doorway. You always want to set yourself up to succeed. Think of each new location as a brand new exercise and proceed through the steps of the stay in each place.

LEAVING YOUR DOG
Power Chair

Remember that your dog is used to moving every time you click the motor on your chair. He either expects to go beside you or he needs to get out of the way. That's why stay is more difficult to teach from a wheelchair. It will take more patience on your part and perhaps more time. Any time you roll over your dog, you need to express your sympathy in a high-pitched, happy voice. If you coddle your dog, it will only reinforce his fear of the wheelchair. Unless he's really hurt, he will snap out of it much faster if you don't give him reason to continue crying. And you'll know if he's really hurt.

Command your dog to sit. Give appropriate praise. Command "stay." Be sure to check your dog's position before you touch your controls. If he is too close for you to move, release him from the stay and try again. It's important that there be no contact between your dog and your wheelchair. If there is, you must be understanding if your dog gets out of the way.

When he's positioned so you won't touch him with the chair, command "stay," and click the control. You want it to make the noise, but you don't want to actually move. The noise itself is enough of a distraction to your dog. Repeat the command "stay" as you click the motor, and quietly praise—"good stay"—then release him. This step may take from a few minutes to a few weeks. You must continue this step until there is absolutely no response from your dog when you click the motor. Remember, you have not moved away from your dog even an inch; you are just getting him used to not moving when he hears the motor if he has heard the stay command first.

When your dog is reliably staying even when he hears the motor click, you will actually move away. Go only an inch or two forward, angling away from your dog. Come right back. Repeat the stay command as you move away and as you return. Your dog may be intimidated by the chair coming at him (although you have hardly moved), and he is apt to pop up. Be ready to repeat the sit and stay commands, firmly but not loudly.

Keep practicing this until you can stay those few inches away for one minute, and until he does not flinch when you return beside him. This, too, may take from a few days to several weeks. Increase the time slowly. If you do it right and don't rush, each step will occur more quickly. Your dog is understanding what you want. Remember to praise, using the words "good stay," while you're away from him.

Now go forward a few feet, angling to the side away from your dog. Immediately back up beside him. Repeat the stay command. Be very careful not to run over any part of your dog as you return. Quietly praise and release. Build up to one minute.

Now go forward about four feet and turn your chair at a right angle to him. Be careful that the leash doesn't pull tight as you go forward.

Don't hesitate to repeat the stay command and/or signal when you face him. (If you've been able to use the hand signal with the stay command, this is when it becomes most helpful. You can simply point your hand, palm first, at your dog as the reminder to stay.) Count to yourself to ten and return beside him. Again, don't hesitate to repeat the stay as you return to him. Quietly praise and release.

If he shifts position to avoid the wheels as you leave him but doesn't move out of the sit, give the command again as a reminder and praise "good stay." If he seems leery of the wheelchair as you return to him, practice by rolling toward him very slowly as you remind him to stay and praise quietly.

Next, command your dog to stay, go forward at least four feet and turn to face him. Some wheelchairs have footrests that stick out a foot or more from the chair. Be sure that there is no danger of the footrests hitting him when you turn to face him. That's why you turn at a right angle to your dog first. You can gauge the distance. If you have protruding footrests, go farther away before you turn to face him.

The other thing you need to be aware of when leaving your dog is that the leash should never pull tight. This would be an unfair signal to him. He must decide whether to obey the stay command or the tug on the leash. Before you leave him, be sure you have enough slack and be careful that it doesn't get caught in the wheels or the footrests.

At each of these stages, practice sometimes in sit and sometimes in down so your dog will learn to stay in any position.

When he is staying reliably when you turn to face him, begin to build up the time that you leave him in this position. A dog can easily stay in a sit for several minutes and a down for half an hour or more. Practice stay in different locations and for varying lengths of time, but remember to be aware of circumstances. Don't expect your dog to sit stay on a slippery floor or on top of an anthill. Don't put him in a down stay in a busy doorway. You always want to set yourself up to succeed. Think of each new location as a brand new exercise and proceed through the steps of the stay in each place.

CHAPTER 11

STAND
Teach Your Dog to Stand on Command

Savannah was lying down next to Blake as he checked out of his health club, but she suddenly got up and ran across the lobby. There she stopped next to a toddler who had just fallen as he waddled into the area. She stood perfectly still beside him, as if he had given her a "stand" command, while he grabbed onto her to help himself stand up. Then he leaned on her sturdy shoulders for balance until his Mom came and picked him up.

WHAT IS STAND?

It's fairly obvious that stand means to stand on all four feet, and your dog does this all the time. But you will need to teach him to do it when you tell him to and to hold the position for as long as you need it.

You might not see any specific need for having your dog stand, but it can be a very helpful exercise. If you groom your dog, having him stand calmly while you brush him can be a big help. When you take him to the vet, if you can command "stand," it will make it much easier for your vet to do the examination. Plus, it can help calm a nervous dog to concentrate on obeying your commands while the vet touches him.

If you intend to train your dog to be a service dog, one helpful exercise you might want to teach is "brace." Your dog will learn to let you gently lean on him so you can get up from a chair or the floor. It may be that stand is the best position for your dog to be in. If he already knows the stand command when you start teaching brace, it will go much faster.

TEACHING STAND

Although dogs stand around all the time, teaching him to stand on command and in one position may take some time. Your dog has learned to sit and lie down on command, and he's very quick to sit for a treat. So you'll find that you'll have to use patience, and you may have to be clever to prevent him from sitting.

There are several methods to teach stand and you just need to experiment and find the one that works best for you and your dog.

The key is to get him off his butt, so you may want to try walking him forward a step or two and then command "stand." As soon as you stop moving, he will probably try to sit, so if possible, slip your hand under his belly, just in front of his back legs. If your dog is sensitive, he may shy away from this. If you can get your hand in there, just gently prevent him from sitting, while you say, "good stand." Wait only a second or two, remove your hand and release him.

If it's difficult for you to move forward, you can hold a piece of food

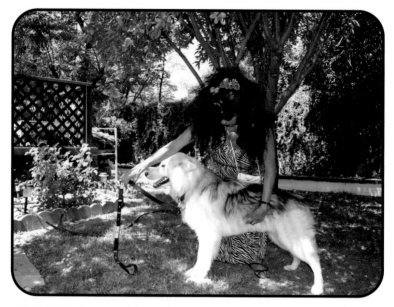

Pull the leash straight forward, not up or down, and place your hand on your dog's flank to help him learn the stand. Betty Wittels (arthrogryposis) and Tikaani (husky mix)

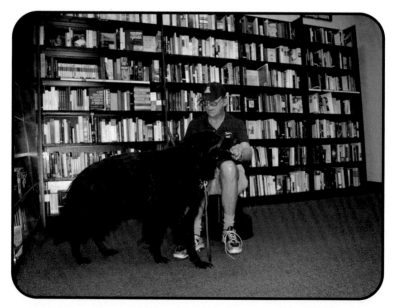

Holding a piece of food straight out will entice your dog to stand up. Bob Ruskin (Parkinson's disease and epilepsy) and Calypso (Belgian sheepdog)

in front of his nose and move it straight out away from him. Don't raise it up or he will sit for it. Move it out in a straight line from his nose. As he stands up to follow the food, say his name and "stand." Praise, "good stand," and give him the treat while he's standing. Then quickly release.

If your dog is small, you can gently lift up his rear end as you say his name and "stand." Keep your hand on his flank and praise "good stand." As soon as you remove your hand, he will probably sit, so you want to be sure and give him the release command first.

If you can't bend over, it may be easier to have your dog up on a raised surface, just as you taught the down command. Once he's up on the sofa, use food to entice him to stand up, and place your hand gently under his flank. Say his name and the command, and praise—"good stand"—while he is standing up. Release him after only a few seconds.

Whatever method, or combination of methods, you try, remember that he will not know what you're asking him to do at first. You must be consistent. Don't wait to praise him until he has sat down; he needs to hear praise while he's standing. Only ask for a few seconds before you release him.

Practice faithfully for at least a week. He should be beginning to get the idea that this word has a specific meaning. Now, command "stand" and see if he has any response. If he starts to get up, encourage him. Hold a treat out in front of him to show him the position you want. If he makes no move at all, then just continue to practice as you've been doing. He needs more time. Make sure you give the command, and make sure you praise when he's in the correct position.

There are a lot of things you're trying to do all at once, and you need to concentrate on doing them correctly for your dog to learn this command. If you tug upward on the leash, your dog will probably sit, so be sure any leash movement is straight forward. If you raise your hand holding the treat, he will sit, and if you lower your hand, he will lie down. So you have to keep your hand on a straight line out from his nose. Remember to say "stand" so he can associate a word with this action, and praise "good stand." But be sure to give the command and the praise as he's standing, not as he's starting to sit. Wait only a second or two, and then give your release word.

If he doesn't seem to be making progress, make sure you're not confusing him with conflicting signals. Be patient. It will take a week or two of diligent practice for him to learn that the word stand has a specific meaning. And it will take months for him to understand it thoroughly and obey it promptly.

PERFECTING THE STAND

It's important to practice stand regularly. Build up the time you ask him to remain in the stand position. If he sits before you release him, put him back in the stand. Put your hand gently under his belly, if you're able to, just as a reminder to stay on all fours. Praise quietly as you gently stroke his belly. Wait several seconds, as you continue to tell him "good stand." Then release him. Sometimes, instead of releasing him, you can give him another command, like sit or down. Be sure to praise when he obeys each command.

When he's readily obeying the stand command, take your hand away from under his belly. Continue to praise "good stand," so he knows he's supposed to remain in position. If he sits when you take your hand away, then he doesn't know the stand command yet and you need to practice longer. If he remains in the stand position, give appropriate praise and then release him.

Now, command "stand." Praise when he stands. Command "stay" just as you did with sit and down. Use your hand signal in front of his face, if you're able, which will remind him what the command means. If he starts to move or sit down, say "uh-uh-uh," and repeat "stand, stay." After a few seconds, praise and release.

Now it's just a matter of building up time on the stand stay as you did for sit and down stays. Build up slowly. Rather than moving away from your dog, concentrate on stand stay with you right next to him. Practice longer and longer times for the stand stay but don't worry about distance. Most of your uses for the stand will require you to be right there with your dog.

When he will maintain a stand stay for at least thirty seconds, have a friend come up and pet him while he holds the position. If he moves to greet the person, use your verbal correction and a firm reminder that he's on a stand and a stay. Your friend should move back while you reposition your dog. Then try again. It may take many tries, but he will learn to remain in the stand position while being touched by a person.

Practice with as many different people as you can enlist to help. If your dog is very shy, always work with people he knows and likes. As his confidence grows, you can begin to introduce him to strangers. But work up slowly. If he's more afraid of men, practice with lots of women first. If he's afraid of the vet, work on this command for months at home. Then take him to the vet's office and practice all his obedience in the waiting room. If he's shaking and shivering, don't tell him it's okay, just work patiently and positively on his obedience commands. Having something to concentrate on other than his fear will help him relax.

Do this several times before you actually go in to see the vet. Ultimately you want your dog to maintain a stand stay while being examined by the vet, but that may take a long time to achieve. Work with lots of praise and food, and have the vet give your dog treats. Most vets, although they're quite busy, are happy to cooperate in this kind of training, because it will make their job easier in the long run.

USING THE STAND

Continue to practice stand and stand stay often. If you groom your own dog, this is a great place to use this command. Use treats and lots of praise to get your dog to maintain the stand while you brush him. Most dogs enjoy being brushed, so this will be an added reward for the stand.

When your dog is doing a solid stand stay, you may find other uses for this exercise. Kellie took her German shepherd with her to school and would often use Atlee's broad, strong back to hold a library book while she looked up some information. You can put things in and out of your dog's pack if he's standing quietly beside you. And you can begin to teach him "brace" (taught in TEAMWORK II). This may be a useful exercise to help you rise from a chair, step up a curb, or to transfer from bed to wheelchair. Of course, your dog must be big enough and strong enough for the brace exercise.

Practice this exercise in different places and for varying lengths of time. You may find many other helpful uses for the stand.

CHAPTER 12

RANDOM RECALL
Teach Your Dog to Come to You When You Call

People often think that all commands to a dog must be issued in loud, gruff, serious tones. Mary was trying to teach her first dog, Lucky, to come. She wanted him to know she meant business so her command sounded strict and harsh. Thinking she was mad at him, he slunk in slowly toward her. Mary's helper said, "Pretend he's got a hundred-dollar bill in his mouth." Mary immediately squealed in a delighted tone, "Lucky! Come!" And the little black terrier raced to her in joy.

WHAT IS RANDOM RECALL?

In our context, recall means your dog will come to you when called, and random means that he will come no matter where he is and no matter what he's doing. Your dog will learn that coming to you is more important and more pleasurable than any distraction.

This means that coming to you must always be rewarded. You must never call your dog to you and then yell at him. No matter how angry you are with your dog, if you call him and he comes to you, you must praise him profusely. If he hates baths or grooming, don't call him to you and immediately clip his nails or put him in the tub. Reward him for coming, pet him and talk to him for a few minutes, then bathe or groom him.

The other important thing to remember about the recall is not to call your dog with the "come" command if you're not in a position to enforce the command. If your dog is running through the woods or chasing a cat, don't yell "Come" in the early stages of training and expect him to obey the command. You would be teaching him that "come" really means go on chasing the cat. Use a whistle, clap your hands, run the other way, or fall down on the ground. Any of these will be more effective than the word come until your dog really knows what come means. Try to avoid any situation where your dog gets away from you until he is reliable on the recall. If he does get away, don't say "come" or he will quickly learn that the word doesn't have any power.

TEACHING RANDOM RECALL

Food is the prime motivator for the recall. You will use the dog's natural instinct to come for food. Remember to praise enthusiastically every time he obeys.

Begin by using your dog's feeding as a training tool. As you go into the kitchen (or wherever you feed him) say his name and "come" in a happy voice. As you get his food out, even though he's right there with you, say his name and "come" in a happy voice. As soon as he looks at you, give appropriate praise. This is not a command; you are just building a positive association with the word you will use as the command.

Do this for a week. Say his name and "come" using a high, happy voice every time you feed your dog even though he is right there with you. Now, sneak away, if you can, while he's sleeping. Go to the place where you normally feed your dog and get a piece of food. Rattle the bag or dog-cookie box and call him. Using a high, happy voice, say his name and "come" in an excited way. He should come running. Give enthusiastic praise and the food treat.

If you're unable to sneak away from your dog—many dogs are so tuned into your every move, especially the sound of a power chair—have a friend pet and distract him while you go to his feeding spot. The second that you call your dog, your friend must immediately release him so he can come to you right away. Praise happily and give a food reward.

You want to be sure you have him under your control when he comes, so command him to sit when he gets to you. You don't want him to think that he can run on past you. You must decide the place you want him to sit—right in front of you or one side or the other, facing either towards you or the same direction you're facing. It's your choice.

Decide where the best spot is and then use the food to get your dog there. As soon as he comes to you, praise for the recall, but move your hand with the food treat to the place where you want him to go. As soon as he's there, tell him "sit." Give appropriate praise and the food as soon as he sits.

Make this a part of your recall from now on. Remember to praise separately for the recall and the sit. Don't wait until he sits for him to hear praise. Sometimes have two food treats in your hand—one for coming, then the other when he sits. It will not take very long for your dog to go automatically to the spot you have designated every time he comes to you.

Practice this for a week, then go to another room and call him. Use that high, happy voice and encourage him to come and find you. If you live in a house with a lot of rooms, begin in the same room as your dog, then move to an adjacent room.

Praise your dog as he's coming to you. Remember that you're teaching him to want to come to you more than he wants to do whatever it was he was just doing. As soon as he has come to you, praise in a very happy voice, then give the food treat. Make sure he

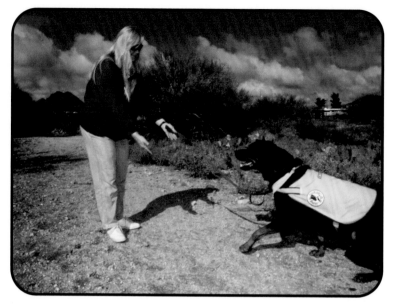

Take plenty of time practicing recalls on leash with enticing body language, enthusiastic praise and tempting food reward. Kim Swingle (degenerative disc disease & arthritis) and Xanth (rottweiler)

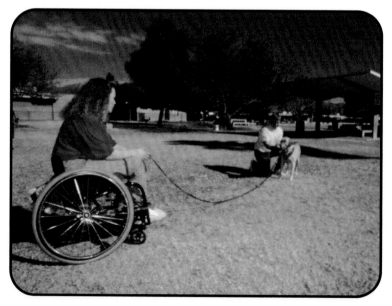

Practicing long line recalls in the park, a friend can hold your dog until you are ready to call him. Helen gets help from husband, Leo. Helen Enfield (spinal cord injury T 6-7) and Nutmeg (yellow lab)

sits in "his spot."

Dogs love to play hide and seek. You're working with this natural fun instinct. Make sure that he can find you easily at first. You can gradually make it more difficult, but always make it fun. Always let him succeed. Remember to continue to call and encourage your dog all the way to you.

Within a short time, your dog will come running whenever you call him. It's a positive and happy experience. What you want is a dog that doesn't even have to think about whether he will respond to the command or not. It's such a positive association that simply hearing the word come causes an immediate and totally automatic response. Remember to give enthusiastic praise as soon as he gets to you and remember to give the praise before the food reward. Get your dog to sit each time.

Next, begin to taper off on the food. Always praise profusely, but leave out the food reward every fourth recall, then every third. Then give food treats randomly. Sometimes do three or four in a row with no treat, then three or four in a row with a treat every time. You want your dog to hope there will be food in it for him, but you want him willing and happy to come with or without food. That's why your praise must be enthusiastic.

PERFECTING THE RECALL

When you know your dog is coming to you quickly and happily every time you call him inside the house, you can start to practice the random recall in other places. Begin in your fenced backyard. Treat it like starting a new exercise. Give food every time for at least a week. At first you want a quiet environment for teaching, so don't have distractions such as children or other pets in the yard. As your dog gets more and more responsive, you can bring in distractions.

As soon as your dog moves away from you in the backyard, say his name and "come" in that happy, high-pitched voice. Use your attention signal and encourage him to respond, but don't give come as a command. Keep your voice upbeat and happy. If your dog doesn't come, it means he doesn't really know what you want. You must go back inside and start all over again.

If he does come, give enthusiastic praise and a food reward. You may need to remind him where he's supposed to sit. Use food to get him to the proper position and praise enthusiastically. Then give him his release word which means he's free to do whatever he wants. When he wanders away, wait a few minutes before you call him again. You don't want him to think you're nagging him. Just move casually around in your yard and take two or three opportunities to call him.

Remember that your tone of voice is still making this a game. Your praise must be very enthusiastic, and it must come before the food treat.

If your dog won't leave your side, get a friend to pet and distract him while you move a few feet away. As soon as you call him, your friend must stop petting or holding him so he can come to you without resistance.

Build up the recalls the same way you did inside. Remember that "slow is fast." The longer you take perfecting the recall in a controlled environment, the more confidence you will have calling him in any situation.

LIFESAVER

The recall can save your dog's life. If he gets away from you, there are all kinds of dangers he might find. If he learns that coming to you is always better and more positive than whatever has distracted him, he will respond to your command instantly, and that instant may be the difference between getting hit by a car, being sprayed by a skunk, or falling off a ledge. The association with the word come must always be a positive one. Remember that as you begin working on recalls in an open area.

Go to a quiet park and check out the area for distractions such as dogs and children. Have your dog on a long line. It's easiest to use a retractable leash which reels in the slack automatically, but any long line will do. Just be careful that it doesn't get tangled on anything. Have your food reward ready before you call him.

Give him a release, so he knows he's not on a heel or any other command. If he wanders away, give him some slack in the line. As soon as he is just a few feet away from you, call him in that happy voice. If he looks at you, praise him and encourage him to come in.

If he doesn't come, give a gentle tug on the leash and call him with enthusiasm. Give happy praise as soon as he gets to you, followed by the food treat. He should go automatically to "his spot" near you and sit. If he doesn't, move the food to that spot and command "sit." But remember to praise for the recall and the sit separately.

Release him and give him some slack. Move around with him and let him sniff and explore. Then call him again. Do this two or three times and then go home. When you call him to you for that last time and head for the car or home, make it very positive. Don't let him think it means his fun is all over. Make leaving the park a happy experience. Use a happy tone of voice to convey to him that the fun is just starting. You don't want him ever to think that coming to you means the good part is over.

As you practice more and more recalls, begin to call him from longer distances. Have a friend hold him and go all the way to the end of your long line. He should still be on leash so that if he decides that some distraction is more interesting than you are, you can correct him with a tug on the leash. Always praise him profusely when he comes.

When you've been practicing recalls in the park for at least a month, and your dog always comes to you quickly and eagerly, you should try an off-leash recall. This is only because your dog might sometime get loose; it's not safe to make a habit of having your dog off leash.

Make sure there are no distractions that will make this a negative experience. Make sure he knows you have the food ready. Have a friend hold and pet your dog while you go no farther than six feet away. Call your dog and encourage him all the way in. Give praise for the recall and command him to sit if he doesn't automatically. He should get food one hundred percent of the time when practicing off-leash recalls, but always remember to praise first.

You are only practicing off-leash recalls to give yourself confidence that your dog will come in an emergency. If at any time you call your dog and he doesn't come, don't get angry or panicked. Don't chase him. Keep a high-pitched, happy tone of voice, encouraging him to look at you. Say "goodbye," then turn and go the opposite direction. This is especially effective in a power chair. If

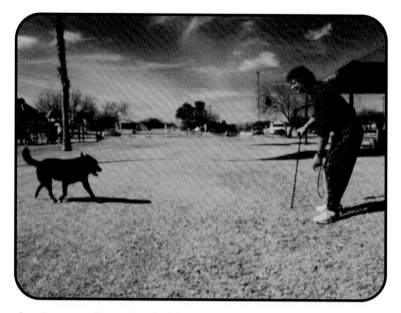

Any time you call your dog, do things to make yourself more inviting, such as bending down and encouraging him. Glenn Rosenberg (spinal cord injury incomplete L 5) and Louis (lab/border collie)

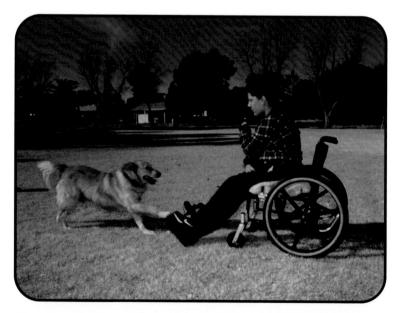

The end result of lots of practice is a dog who comes quickly and eagerly in response to your call. Stephen Krause (arthrogryposis) and Jake (golden retriever)

you can bend down and make yourself inviting, do so. Don't get annoyed; your dog will hear that in your voice and hesitate even more. When he does finally come to you, you must praise him as if nothing happened.

DOG PARKS

It can be counter-productive for people with disabilities to allow their dogs to run loose and play with other dogs in the park. It may encourage him to pull during the heel, which could cause you to fall. It may give your dog the idea that he is in control and that you can't enforce commands like "come" and "heel." You're much better off playing with him in your backyard and taking long walks with him on leash. He will find these controlled activities enjoyable and your relationship will be strengthened.

But more and more dog parks are springing up everywhere. They are wonderful fenced-in areas where dogs can be off leash and still be safe. However, you must have good control of your dog in order to use a dog park. Work on basic obedience commands as you approach the enclosure. If your dog pulls and won't listen to you, turn away until you gain control. If you follow through and insist on his obedience, he will settle down. Soon he will learn that being able to run and play in the dog park is his reward for obeying your commands. Use treats and lots of praise. Once you get inside the enclosure and he's enjoying the other dogs, occasionally call him to you, making sure he knows you have lots of good food rewards for him.

It's great for dogs to be able to run and play together, but you must maintain control of your dog. Also be aware of the other dogs in the enclosure. If your dog is shy, he may be overwhelmed by more dominant dogs. Keep a close eye on the activity and be ready to leave if it becomes too much for him. If your dog is dominant, make sure he doesn't bully other dogs. Again, be ready to leave if he becomes too much for the other dogs.

Using places like dog parks to practice obedience will help solidify the training. Don't nag your dog with constant work—he needs time to play—just make sure you have control of your dog and the situation.

An alternative is to set up a "play date" with a friend and their dog at your house or theirs. You can watch the dogs interact and learn more about their body language and breed characteristics. It's fun, totally controlled, and educational.

CHAPTER 13

CONTROLLED WALK
Teach Your Dog to Walk Beside You under Control

Training an older dog can be a challenge, especially if the dog has been spoiled. Margaret doted on her 5-year-old toy poodle and was having trouble teaching her to walk on the leash. The instructor was trying to keep the class moving while explaining to Margaret how to encourage her dog to walk beside her. The other students in class were doing well, and Margaret's frustration became apparent when the instructor told the class, "Forward." Margaret looked at everyone walking away, picked up her dog in her arms, and marched resolutely with the rest of the class.

WHAT IS CONTROLLED WALK?

Traditionally, in obedience training, a person and dog walking together is called "heeling." It's a very formal, structured exercise with the person walking a certain way and the dog on the left side in a "proper heel position." If you wish to show your dog in obedience competition, you must learn to do this exercise that formal way. But for you and your dog to be able to go places together in a casual yet controlled manner, we simply want you to learn a "controlled walk."

The controlled walk is when your dog is walking beside you with slack in the leash. If he is pulling or weaving or sniffing the ground constantly, he may be walking, but he is not controlled. The goal of this exercise is to get him to learn to walk at your side calmly and at your pace, to stop when you stop, to turn when you turn.

It doesn't matter which side your dog walks on, but choose one and stick with it. Traditionally in dog training, dogs have been taught to heel on the left, but there is no practical reason behind it. If you prefer or need him to be on your right, then that is where he should walk. It may be to your personal advantage to have him walk a little ahead or a little behind. Again, that's your choice. You simply have to decide the proper heel position for you and then teach it to your dog. But you are the one to decide, not him.

You are also the one who decides the pace. Dogs naturally prefer to move rapidly. If you are in a wheelchair and can move along at a quick pace, this will be an advantage, but if you walk slowly your dog will learn to adjust. It will just require more patience.

The parts of the controlled walk include starting, walking, and stopping. Each must be understood and practiced in order to achieve a smooth controlled walk.

STARTING

Traditionally, the command given is "heel," but any word or phrase will do. Some people say, "walk with me" or "let's go." Whatever you choose, remember to give the command as you begin to move. Don't start off and then say "heel." Your dog is not a mind reader; he needs to be told whether you expect him to stay put or to move with you. The idea is to begin together smoothly.

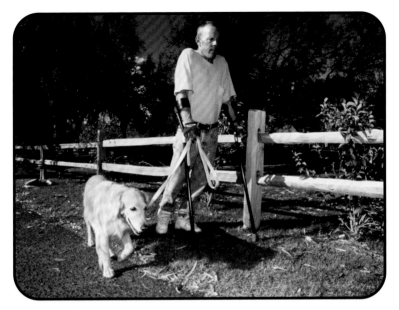

A dog might walk wide of the crutches, especially during the early stages of training. Blake Gigli (spinal cord injury T 12) and Savannah (golden retriever)

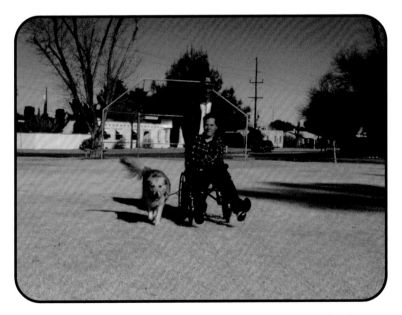

Sometimes it's necessary to receive assistance while teaching the controlled walk. Steve's dad, Jon, helps by pushing the chair. Stephen Krause (arthrogryposis) and Jake (golden retriever)

WALKING

You proceed at your own pace and your dog is the one to make the adjustments. He learns to pay attention to you so that he will turn when you turn. He will walk close enough to you so that his leash doesn't get caught on anything, like street signs or people, but not so close that he crowds you.

Talk to him to keep his attention and praise "good heel," "good walk." It's important to keep your tone of voice upbeat and happy. If words are difficult for you, happy sounds will do. What you say is completely unimportant; he will be listening to the happy tone of voice and responding in a positive manner.

STOPPING

It's important that when you stop for any reason, your dog stops promptly too. If you want to teach him to sit automatically, give him a "sit" command each time you stop. If you prefer him to stand beside you when you stop, use a "wait" or "stop" command rather than "sit." The important thing is that he stops next to you and waits for the next command.

TEACHING THE CONTROLLED WALK

This is the first time that you have asked your dog to move along beside you. You began by teaching him the control commands—sit, down, stand, and stay. Then you taught him to come to you. Now he must learn to move with you and at your pace. Don't expect him to automatically understand what you're asking him to do.

Begin in a quiet area without any distractions—inside your house or your own backyard. It's important that you have your dog's attention, so children and other pets should not be running around while you're working. You want to build up positives and set him up to succeed, so begin teaching heel in an area where you will have your dog's undivided attention.

If you sometimes walk and sometimes use a wheelchair, you'll want to practice heeling both ways. Your pace will be different, and your dog must learn to make the proper adjustments. You may have better control from the wheelchair, so you might want to start out that way. When your dog has learned what heel means and he's

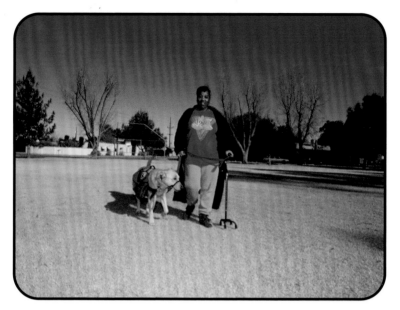

The head halter may give you much better control when walking your dog
in the park. Nadine Snyder (lupus and multiple sclerosis) and
Blondy (yellow lab)

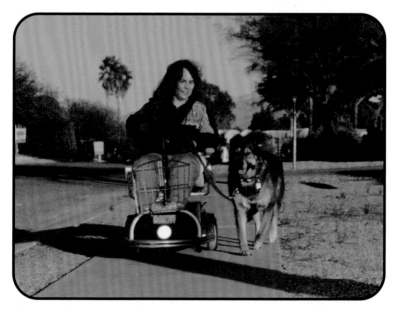

Once taught the proper position and pace, your dog will walk beside you on
a nice loose leash. Annette Stone (multiple sclerosis) and
Bandit (shepherd mix)

walking beside you under good control, you can practice on foot.

To begin, you should go only a short distance. Your dog doesn't instinctively know what position or pace you want; you will have to teach him. That means you won't adjust to his pace but will teach him to adjust to yours.

Before you move, say your dog's name and "heel" or whatever word or signal you choose, and move forward. If he doesn't come right with you, give a gentle tug on the leash and repeat the command. If he leaps ahead of you, stop immediately and command him to sit or stop. Praise for the stop. Then, after repeating your heel command, move forward again.

It may take several starts and stops for your dog to know what you mean. He will get tired of stopping and being made to sit or stop every time he leaps forward and will eventually move under more restraint. As soon as he is walking beside you, even if it's only for a step or two, praise, "good heel." If he then bolts ahead, stop and command him to sit or stop.

The idea is to correct him for the behavior you don't want (leaping ahead and pulling) and to praise him for what you do want (walking by your side). As with all commands, it will take patience and consistency on your part for him to understand the difference.

If you are using the traditional training collar, it's very important that you use it correctly in heeling. If it's tight all the time, you are not communicating properly with your dog. You must give the "jerk and release" as explained in "Equipment" (page 45). If you're using a head halter, you just need to remember to give slack when he is in the proper position.

If your dog tends to lag—walk behind you, not wanting to keep up—your praise and enthusiasm are even more important while teaching controlled walk. If you can hold a piece of food while moving, you may find this helpful with a dog who lags. If you are unable to hold food, you will have to make your praise reward enough. Do very short sessions of straight-line heeling. Keep your voice light and happy, and praise with enthusiasm every time he is beside you. You will need patience to work with a dog who lags, so remember to encourage with positive, happy tones.

POSITION

You must decide the correct position for your dog. It should be whatever works best for you, but remember that a dog will naturally heel a little wider beside crutches or a wheelchair. You choose the best position and then teach it to him. Don't allow him to wander, sometimes ahead, sometimes behind. Correct him when he's out of position, and praise him when he's in the right place.

Be careful with crutches and wheelchairs that the leash doesn't get tangled and give an unfair correction. You should have only enough slack in the leash for your dog to walk in the place you have chosen as "heel position." You may want to mark the leash with a knot or a second loop in the place you want to hold it.

One of the difficulties in a manual wheelchair is that you pull your arms back to grip the back of the wheels and then roll forward. What this may do is give a leash correction to your dog with every back motion, even if he is in proper position. You must be sure there is enough slack in the leash for your backward stroke, but not enough to get tangled in the wheel.

TURNS

After you've practiced several sessions of short, straight-line heeling, begin to practice turning and walking around obstacles to teach your dog to pay attention to you while walking. Talk to him. Tell him you're going to turn. Don't do military-type turns. Gentle gradual changes of direction are best. You might want to use commands, like "right" and "left" which he will eventually learn and be able to recognize. Give your dog lots of warning and make sure he's under control before you turn.

If you use crutches, they can be a valuable training tool as long as they are used gently. As you get ready to turn, you may put the crutch in front of your dog if he's too far ahead of you, and praise immediately when he's back beside you. You may push very lightly with the crutch if your dog crowds you, but never use them in a way that might make him afraid of them.

You have an advantage practicing turns from a manual or power chair. You can use your chair as a training tool. To teach him to watch you, turn quickly in either direction. You need to be careful

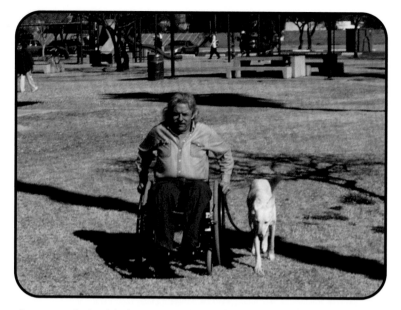

In a manual wheelchair, you must be careful not to pull the leash tight on the back stroke. Mike Landwehr (spina bifida) allows plenty of slack for Ruby (white shepherd mix).

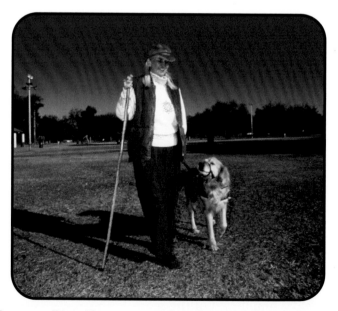

Whatever walking aid you use, your dog will learn to pay attention to you and go at your pace if you practice with diligence and consistency. Lynn Koons (Charcot Marie Tooth) and Mr. Darcy (golden retriever)

not to run over him, but he will soon learn to pay attention while walking beside you if the wheelchair suddenly comes at him or spins away from him. You can use the weight of the wheelchair to help you make a correction. All of your practice should be in a positive manner—don't make your dog afraid of your crutches or your chair. Remember that if you should accidentally hit your dog, don't baby him. Express your apology in a happy, high pitched tone, and keep going. Above all, your dog must hear lots of appropriate praise when he is walking correctly beside you.

PERFECTING THE CONTROLLED WALK

After several short sessions, you and your dog should be able to walk together under fairly good control. It will take a long time to get total control and will require patience and practice on your part. You must be consistent. If you slack off in what you expect your dog to do, he will get sloppy. Whenever you command "heel," he must remain in that heel position. Give him a release if you want to let him wander to the end of the leash. If he's under heel command, he should not go to greet another dog or a person. Always get him under control and then release him from the heel command to go visit. This is especially important for a service dog who is expected to function well in crowded malls and restaurants. Set the standards now and stick to them. You will have a much easier time later if you do.

As your dog gets under more and more control, move out of your safe environment and try heeling in different places. Go to the park but expect major distractions and be prepared to deal with them consistently. If your dog gets away from you to play with another dog in the park, you will have twice the difficulty the next time you go. Take him to a quiet park first and build up the positives before you go to the more crowded park.

If you want to let him run and play in a dog park, be sure you keep him under control until you get in the enclosure. Make him heel up to the fence, and if he won't heel properly, turn away and continue to practice heel. He must learn to pay attention to you and obey you, even though he really wants to run and play. When you are inside the enclosure and he is calm and under control, take off his leash and give him either the release word or a specific command to play. Always give this command to keep you in charge of the situation.

Proceed slowly with the heel exercise. If your dog is young and enthusiastic, or shy and fearful, take the time to build up his confidence and composure. Be aware of the distractions and how they might affect him. A dog that walks calmly and under control beside you is a joy to take everywhere. Remember: "Slow is fast."

CHAPTER 14

WAIT
Teach Your Dog to Wait at Doors

Colonel was a well-trained retriever. He had titles from dog shows and field trials, and was an exceptionally obedient dog. His owner, Jack, came home from shopping and found Colonel sitting stiffly in the middle of the living room obviously uncomfortable. He called his dog over, and Colonel promptly and proudly came. Jack couldn't find anything wrong nor could he figure out Colonel's behavior. It happened again the next day. The mystery was cleared up a few days later when Jack, from the kitchen, heard the parrot issue a very commanding, "Colonel, STAY!"

THE WAIT EXERCISE

What is the "wait" exercise and how is it different from "stay"? When you command your dog to stay, you mean that he must not move from the place or the position that you left him until released or given another command. If you leave him in a sit stay, he must not lie down or move forward, but must remain in the sit position exactly where you left him.

There are many times when you don't want your dog to leave a certain area, but it's not necessary that he remain in one position. When you leave home, for instance, you don't expect your dog to remain motionless by the door until you return. Yet many people tell their dogs to stay as they leave the house. You don't really mean stay and your dog knows you don't really mean it. He doesn't stay motionless by the door, and that may undermine the times when you really do want him to stay. For the times when you don't really mean stay, you need another command. This is when you use wait.

What wait really means is that you have erected an invisible barrier that your dog cannot cross until you give him permission. If you don't want your dog in the kitchen you'll use wait, which will come to mean that he can move around as much as he wants in the living room, but he can't cross into the kitchen.

You must teach him that all doors to the outside, as well as gates from the yard have "wait barriers." Your dog will learn to wait for your permission. Opening the car door is not license for him to jump out. He must learn to wait until you give the release word.

Wait is a life-saving command. Aside from demonstrating good manners and excellent control, it can keep your dog from running out of your house into the street or jumping out of a car into traffic.

TEACHING WAIT

As critical as wait is for your dog to know, it's one of the easier commands to teach, but like all commands, you have to be consistent in your approach. Even if your dog has always run out the door or jumped out of the car, decide that from now on he will wait for permission. That means every time. You must not let him get away with slipping out. You must control the situations.

Don't open your front door unless your dog is on leash and by your side. Don't assume that just because he's in another room that he won't hear you open the door and come running. If he slips past you out the door, he's been rewarded for incorrect behavior. Don't give the wait command unless you know you can keep him from bolting out the door.

"Wait" does not have to be the word you use for the command. Whether it's verbal or a signal, be certain that it's different from your stay command.

You must decide where the barrier is. You need to get a mental picture of how far your dog can go and what line he cannot cross. Then stick with it. If you allow him to put one foot out the door today, tomorrow he may put two, and the next day he may bolt out.

WAIT AT AN OPEN DOOR

Put your dog on leash and give the wait command before you open the door. You want to open the door slightly or have a friend open it. You command "wait," then shut the door firmly.

If your dog backs away from the slamming door, give appropriate praise. Repeat the sequence, opening the door a little farther this time. If he tries to go out, use the leash or your wheelchair to prevent him. Be careful not to close the door on his head, and be sure to praise when he backs up.

Most dogs don't like having a door slammed in their face. It's amazing how fast this technique works. Do this several times a day for several days. You should begin to see your dog backing up as you give the wait command, not waiting for the door to be slammed. This means he is learning the word.

Now open the door all the way. Remember to give the command before you open the door. Have your dog on leash beside you and go up to the doorway. Stop wherever you decide your dog's barrier is. Usually it's the doorjamb that you don't want him to cross without permission. As soon as he is at the barrier, give the wait command again. Use a firm tone of voice or an emphatic signal to convey that you mean it.

If he stops or backs up, praise, "good wait." If he tries to go out, use the leash to stop him. If you're in a wheelchair, back up and pull your dog back with you or block the doorway with your chair. Do whatever you need to do to make sure he doesn't go past your barrier.

If this step is a struggle, you haven't spent enough time teaching him the meaning of the command "wait." Go back to opening the door and slamming it until he responds to the command itself, not just the door slam.

Be aware of distractions outside when you approach the open door. It may be too much for your dog if the neighbor's cat is sunning himself on your front lawn. Keep temptations to a minimum during the early training stages. You can bring in distractions later, but at the beginning, you always want to succeed in a positive manner.

There are two things your dog must learn to do at an open front door. He must learn to wait and then go out with you on your command and under your control, and he must learn that there are times when he will not be permitted to go out at all.

When he is waiting beside you without trying to escape, praise him: "Good wait." Then give either your release word or a command to go out. You and your dog should go out the door together, under control. If he tends to leap out ahead of you, give him the "heel" command so he knows he is still working.

If you're in a wheelchair you probably need him to get behind you in order to fit through the door. Use a command like "back" or "behind." You can use that in any tight spot when there isn't enough room for both of you side by side.

Your dog also needs to know that sometimes you will go out the door and he won't be allowed to. When he is doing a very solid wait beside you, repeat the wait command as you go through the doorway. Use your body or your chair to block him if he tries to come with you. Give the wait command very firmly. Praise—"good wait"—if he stops or backs up. Praise quietly so he doesn't take it as an invitation to join you.

You should go just barely out the door, praise, and then come right back beside him. Praise and release by moving away from the door into the house. Don't let him take the opportunity to bolt out the door.

You may need help in teaching this, especially if you're in a wheelchair. It's difficult for you to see what your dog is doing as you're going out the door. Have a friend stand behind your dog and hold the leash. If he tries to follow you out the door, your friend can give a tug as you repeat the wait command.

Build up the time and distance that you can leave your dog waiting for you at the open door. Build up very slowly. If he runs outside after a wait command, he has rewarded himself for incorrect behavior, and it will now take longer to correct.

After weeks of practicing faithfully and consistently, you will be able to leave your dog on a wait at an open door for several minutes. You can get groceries from the car or check the mail, and your dog will not run out the door.

The length of time required to teach this exercise thoroughly will vary from dog to dog. If your dog has been running out the door for years, it will take longer than if you're starting with a young dog who never got into this bad habit. But in either case it may be months before the wait is completely solid.

One way you might want to practice wait so that your dog can differentiate between the times he gets to come with you and the times he has to stay home is to back out the door when he has to remain on the wait. This is helpful because you are facing your dog and can see if he starts to follow you. Also your dog will learn that when you back out the door, he doesn't come with you.

Don't hesitate to repeat the wait command firmly if your dog shows signs of coming out. It's a good idea to remind him that he is on a command. It's perfectly okay if he goes into the house, moves from room to room, or lies down on the rug. That's not breaking the wait command. The only thing he can't do is go out the door.

Teach your dog to wait at every door to the outside, and if you have gates, teach him to wait there, too. Every opening to the outside should have a "wait barrier." Each time you move to a new door, treat it like a new exercise. Start at the beginning. You will need to remind him of the rules, but he will learn more quickly each time.

Even when your dog is very good at waiting at the open door, you should always give a wait command whenever the door is opened. Even if your dog is in another room, simply get into the habit of saying "wait" every time you open the door. This also means that

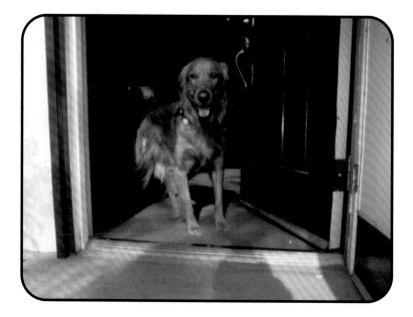

Sedona (golden retriever)

Dogs are taught to "wait" under a variety of circumstances. It's more than just control; it's a matter of safety.

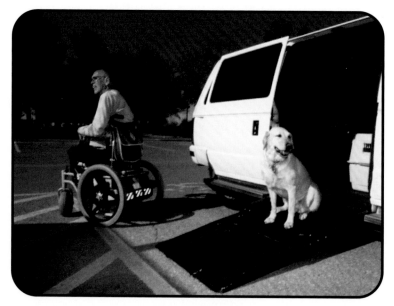

Laura (yellow lab)

when you return to your house, say "wait" firmly as you open the door. Your dog will probably be eagerly waiting for you just inside the door and this will remind him that he can't run out.

WAIT IN THE CAR

Most dogs are very excited to arrive anywhere and as soon as the car is parked they want out. Unless you train him otherwise, your dog will jump out the second a door is opened. He must learn to wait while you get out of the car, until you give him permission to exit. The safest way to transport your dog in a car is either with a seat belt or in a crate. This way, he can't move around and disturb your driving, and he's much safer in an accident. Also, it will make teaching wait in the car easier. Just teach him to wait in the crate until you get his leash attached and give him permission to come out. But if he rides loose in the car, train him to travel calmly and exit the car under control.

If you are physically able, you can practice this very much like wait at the front door. If your dog tends to fly out the first door that's opened, begin by commanding "wait" in a firm tone. Open your door just a crack and then close it. Praise if he backs away from the door—be sure to say "good wait." Open the door a little farther and close it hard. Say "wait" as you open the door and praise as your dog backs away. It may take many repetitions to teach the very excited dog to allow you to get out first.

If you aren't able to open and slam the door yourself, have a friend stand outside and open it as you command "wait." Instruct your friend to open the door only a fraction and then slam it. You give the command and the praise. Build up to the point where the door can be open, you can get out, and your dog will wait. Be very firm in your wait command, especially if your dog makes any move toward the door. Be lavish in your praise when he backs away from the door.

To be certain that your dog will not bolt over you and out the door, you might want to attach his leash to some fixed object in the car. Your dog should not be on a choke collar if you do this. You want to restrain him, not choke him. (In fact, your dog should never have the choke collar or head halter on when the car is moving, nor should his leash be attached. It's too dangerous.)

As soon as you get out of the car, command "wait" and close the door. If you drive a standard car, it's safest if your dog rides in the back seat so you can teach him to always exit from a different door than you do. This way he will learn to wait for you to get out of the car, open his door, and invite him out. This is not appropriate if you use a van and come out on a ramp. Your dog will need to exit from the same door, but he will still learn to wait for your command.

With a car, proceed just as you taught him to wait at the open door. You are now outside the car and your dog is still inside. Give the command "wait," open the door near your dog just a fraction, and quickly close it. Praise if he backs away; repeat the wait command firmly if he moves toward the door. Do this several times, opening the door a bit more each time unless your dog seems about to bolt out. Never let him get close enough to the door that he might get caught in it when it slams. Open it only a fraction until you see him backing off, then open it a fraction more, and keep it at that level until he backs away each time.

Each step may take only one or two times, or it might take twenty. It depends on your dog's history in the car. If you are totally reteaching him after years of jumping out, you must be patient and understanding.

When you can open the car door fully and your dog backs off and doesn't try to jump out, give him a command to exit the car. You can use any word, such as "out" or "let's go." You can use your release word. Just make sure that you give the same command every time that means he can now get out of the car. Hold the leash, and when he jumps out, command him to come to your side and sit. This way, he will always come out under control, regardless of any distraction.

Using a van, you will need to block your dog's exit. Give a firm wait command, and don't allow him to jump out of the van. An excellent way to teach this is to have a friend restrain your dog by holding the leash. This way, there's no chance of him slipping out. Repeat "wait" firmly if he moves toward the door. Praise if he backs up or simply doesn't pull forward. Then give him a release or a command to get out. You should command him to come to your side and sit so he is always under control when he exits.

During the training phase, even if he's only waiting for a second, be sure to give him the command to exit before he jumps out. He needs to learn to always wait for your permission. In time, you will be able to leave the doors open, get something out of your trunk or talk to friends, and your dog will wait in the car until you tell him it's okay to get out.

Don't practice that until your dog demonstrates a solid wait of a minute or more with you positioned right by the door. Before you walk away from an open door always check for distractions. If there's a squirrel your dog can't resist, or a dog coming by, don't expect him to wait.

Remember, as in all training, "slow is fast." You will accomplish much more, much faster, if you build up slowly under positive circumstances. If your dog jumps out and has the fun of chasing a squirrel, he will be more inclined to ignore your wait command the next time.

CHAPTER 15

LEAVE IT
Teach Your Dog Not to Touch Food Except with Your Permission

It can be very dangerous for a dog to eat things off the ground. He has no way of knowing what's bad for him; he only knows that when something smells good, he should eat it. Cheryl, who is blind, was being guided through the park by her dog. The dog devoured an ice cream cone that was on the ground. The ice cream was covered with ants which bit the dog's throat as they were swallowed. Her head and neck swelled, almost to the point of closing her breathing passage; she might have died. In this case, Cheryl became aware of the situation and got her dog to the vet in time.

WHAT IS LEAVE IT?

"Leave it" is a command which means that your dog is not supposed to touch whatever he was about to touch. In the example on the previous page, the woman was at a distinct disadvantage because she could not see what her dog was doing and the dog scooped up the ice cream before she was aware of any movement. But with diligent training, a dog could learn to never eat any food off the ground. If you have your vision, you can prevent him from going after anything on the ground simply by being aware of your surroundings and your dog's body language, and teaching him the leave it command.

TEACHING LEAVE IT

The word you use is unimportant. You should pick one that you will remember quickly and easily because you may have to get the command out suddenly to prevent a dangerous situation. "Leave it," "no," "out," "mine," "don't touch," and "don't bother" are common commands for this exercise.

If you cannot say words, find a sound that comes out deep and gruff. This is a negative command so it shouldn't sound happy. If you cannot make sounds, your signal should be sharp and abrupt. Whatever you choose, remember to be consistent.

Begin by using a food that's not too tempting to your dog. As he becomes more reliable, you will work up to more enticing foods.

It's easiest to teach leave it with help from a friend. Get your dog on leash and by your side. You want to have a little slack in the leash but not very much. Have your friend put a small piece of food two feet in front of you. As your friend places the food on the ground, you command "leave it." If your dog moves toward the food, use the leash to stop him and repeat the command firmly.

If your dog is wearing a training collar, you should use the "jerk and release" as discussed in the "Equipment" chapter (page 45). Don't keep the leash tight. Give him slack and make the correction again if needed. If you are using a head halter, loosen the leash as soon as he stops pulling toward the food. Be ready to tighten up if he moves toward the food again.

You can use your wheelchair to prevent your dog from getting the food. Use the chair to block him as you firmly repeat the command, and praise when he backs away.

It's critically important that your dog not get to the food. If he eats it after you have commanded "leave it," he's been well rewarded for disobeying your command. That's why you must get yourself completely ready for this command before the food is placed. If your dog goes for food on the floor during this training phase and you are not in a position to stop him, it's better not to give the command at all.

When your dog looks away from the food, or puts slack in the leash, praise "good leave it." He might move toward the food again, so be ready to repeat the command sharply and make a leash correction if necessary. Praise when he backs off.

The first time you try this, leave the food down for only a few seconds, just long enough for him to put slack in the leash so you can praise him. Your friend should then pick up the food and put it out of reach. Never give your dog this piece of food as a reward for leave it. You may put it aside and use it as a reward for some other exercise later, but he must learn that when you say "leave it," it means he does not get that food.

Practice this only one time each training session. You need to build up slowly. Work on the leave it two or three times a day with the food placed two feet away.

Slowly increase the time that you leave the food down, based on your dog's reaction. For the chow hound who is used to eating everything off the floor, this step could take several days or even several weeks.

When your dog doesn't fight the leash to get to the food, have your friend place the food only a foot away. Be ready to make a correction if needed and be sure to give a firm leave it command. Praise when your dog allows slack in the leash, then use your attention signal to get him to look at you. Give enthusiastic praise when he does. This is the ultimate "leave it." He will turn away from the food to look at you. If he doesn't look at you, move away from the food with him and get his attention on you. Then praise him.

PERFECTING LEAVE IT

This is such an important command that you want to be very sure your dog responds consistently. That means you must practice it often under controlled conditions before you test your dog when you don't have leash control. Most dogs hear the disapproval in your voice if you give the command correctly, and they want to please you. This is what overcomes their natural desire for the food, so you must give the command firmly each time. Even more importantly, you must give appropriate praise as soon as your dog turns away or stops pulling forward.

As with all commands, "leave it" should not be shouted. You want your dog to obey a quiet-but-firm command. You don't want to call attention to yourself by having to shout at your dog.

Practice for at least a week, two or three times a day, with the food a foot away from your dog. Vary the kind of food you use— sometimes his kibble, sometimes hot dogs or cheese, something very tempting. Remember not to give a food reward for the leave it. Praise enthusiastically, then get him to look at you and praise for attention.

Now place a piece of food on the floor and walk with your dog past it. Give the leave it command as you approach the food, and be ready to make a correction if necessary. If your dog lowers his head toward the food, repeat the command firmly and move away quickly, bringing him with you. Praise as soon as you are away from the food. Praise enthusiastically if your dog obeyed your first leave it command.

Practice this for a week. If your dog always pulls toward the food, perhaps your command is not coming out sternly enough. You want to be sure he knows that there is no room for negotiation here. He is never going to be allowed to have this food. Check with all household members to be sure no one is giving him food without your permission. Also be sure your praise is prompt and enthusiastic when he leaves the food alone.

You may have a tendency to automatically make a leash correction on your dog. This is very common, but it's important that you make sure that he will obey your verbal command. There will be occasions when you won't have him on leash, but you will need him to leave something alone. If he learns to obey the leash correction only, you will not have any control when he is off leash, so you need to concentrate on practicing the leave it using your voice/signal command only.

As you approach the food on the floor, give the leave it command firmly (remember that doesn't mean loudly). Concentrate on keeping the leash loose. Do not automatically tug on the leash as you get near the food, but give him a chance to obey your voice command first.

If he lowers his head toward the food, repeat the command sternly. If he looks away from the food, praise and keep moving. If he doesn't respond to the command, give a correction and move quickly away from the food. Praise as you move away even if you had to make a correction.

You must continue practicing this until your dog consistently ignores the food when you give the leave it command, and a correction is no longer necessary. There is no telling how long this will take, but it's very important to accomplish it.

LEAVE IT MEANS LEAVE IT FOR ANYTHING

The leave it command doesn't just apply to food on the floor in the house. It's easiest to teach the command under controlled circumstances, but once he knows the command, you will find that you'll use it many times a day.

If your dog shows interest in taking your sock outside to play, a leave it command tells him not to touch it. If the neighbor's cat is in your yard as you go out to the car with your dog, a leave it command will remind your dog to pay attention and stay with you. If you go to the park and your dog finds a cache of chicken bones on the ground, a leave it command may save his life. If you're in the mall and you pass by a child eating an ice cream cone, a leave it command will prevent embarrassment or repercussions from an angry parent.

Always be aware of your dog's body posture. You don't have to stare at your dog constantly or monitor the ground in front of him continuously. When you learn awareness of your dog, you will know instantly when he shows extra alertness. His ears perk up, or his body tenses, or there's a slight tug on the leash. Before you even look to see what's out there, give your leave it command, which should immediately cause your dog to turn away from whatever it was. When you have his attention, you can look to see the cat or squirrel that he almost chased.

Staying one step ahead of your dog will save you and your dog in many situations—keep him from pulling you over, prevent him from running into the street, save big vet bills!

FOOD ON TABLES

The leave it command should also be applied to food on tables and counters. Don't leave tempting food even on high kitchen counters when you're not around to correct your dog. The best dog cannot resist a turkey on a platter or a steak thawing. Don't set him up to fail. But you should be able to leave food on the counter while you are working in the kitchen.

To teach him to ignore food on the counter, place something tempting on the counter and pretend to be busy. If you can manage it, have a book ready to bang on the counter, or use the "shake can" mentioned in the "Behavior" chapter (page 31). The idea is to make a loud noise if your dog approaches the food. Praise when he backs off. If your dog is afraid of loud noises, use a light tap on the counter just to redirect his attention. Praise when he looks at you. You might have to do this several different times, but he will learn he cannot take food off the counters.

Your dog also should not steal food from a low table. You want to know that you can have refreshments out for guests and be able to go answer the phone, for instance, and that your dog will not steal any food. There may be times when you'll have guests who won't know what to do if your dog starts to eat the hors d'oeuvres, and you don't want them to have to worry about it.

After your dog has learned what the command leave it means, place a plate of food on a coffee table and give the command. Be ready to make a correction if necessary. This food is at a much closer level so it may seem more tempting, but if he really knows the command, he should leave the food alone when you tell him. If he goes for the food, use the leash or your wheelchair and move away

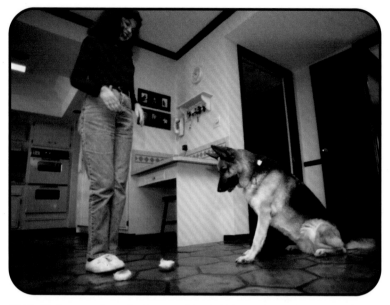

Kellie Christenson (juvenile rheumatoid arthritis) and Atlee (German shepherd)

The "leave it" command means your dog doesn't touch the food whether on the floor or on a low table within easy reach.

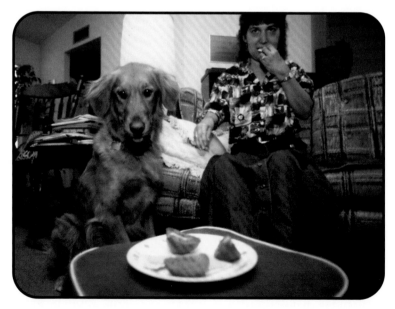

Mary George (rheumatoid arthritis) and Sedona (golden retriever)

from the food quickly.

When your dog is consistently ignoring the food, test to see how trustworthy he is. Have your dog off leash. Put food on the coffee table and have a friend ready to pick up the plate of food if he goes for it. Give the leave it command, and leave the room. If your dog follows you out, it means he will not eat the food. If he stays near the food, he should not touch it.

You shouldn't go far. Praise your dog for not touching the food and come back to remove the temptation. You want to practice this until your dog begins to ignore the food, or at least until you are sure that he won't try to eat it.

CONCLUSION

Leave it is a very important command whether you are training a family pet or a service dog. It's wonderful to have a well-mannered dog who will not touch food and other things when he's told not to. But it's much more than that.

Teaching your dog not to touch something, just because you told him not to, and even though he might really want to, shows him that you are the pack leader; that you have control of the situation. It's not cruel. You aren't starving him. You're simply establishing the rules and sticking to them. Your dog will adjust happily. He will have more respect for you as leader, and this will make everything easier and happier for you both.

CHAPTER 16

AND YOU THOUGHT YOU WERE FINISHED

Now You Can Consider Whether You Would Like to Train Your Dog to the Next Level—Service Dog

Kellie developed juvenile rheumatoid arthritis when she was three years old so she was always known at school as the "kid with arthritis." At age ten, she began training a German shepherd to be her TOP DOG, and by the sixth grade, Atlee was accompanying Kellie to school every day. Suddenly, Kellie was cool—she was the "kid with the dog." Nobody much noticed her arthritis anymore; they were too busy admiring her and her faithful companion. What a positive effect this had on her life!

COMPANION DOG

If you have followed the order and the methods in this book, and if you have worked patiently and consistently with your dog, you now have a well-trained, reliable companion who is easy to live with. You have achieved what very few people are able to accomplish. We know it can be frustrating at times, but we hope the end results make it all worthwhile.

However, it doesn't end here. Even if all you want of your dog is a well-behaved friend at home, you must continue to practice all the exercises. You will find that you will use many of them in your daily interactions with your dog. If he begins to get sloppy on any of them, go back to formal training and remind him that the rules always apply. Whenever you give a command, expect him to obey it. Don't forget to praise him each time he does as you command.

SERVICE DOG

There is much more than basic obedience that your dog can learn. Dogs can be taught any number of skills that can make your life easier. They can pick up almost anything you drop. They can retrieve the telephone, newspaper, your shoes. They can help you get dressed and undressed. They can help you get up out of a chair. They can open and close doors and turn lights on and off. This is only a small sample of the many different things dogs can do to help. In our book, TEAMWORK II, we use the same approach, teaching you how to train your dog to do the specific service exercises that will be useful to you.

A service dog has the same legal rights as a guide dog. A person with a disability may take his service dog almost anywhere he goes—into restaurants, malls, movie theaters, to school or work, onto airplanes. Your responsibility is to have your dog well-prepared and well-trained before you expect the public to welcome him.

IN PUBLIC

Your dog must learn to perform all the basic obedience exercises in public with distractions. You must expose him, slowly and under controlled circumstances, to the kinds of places you will be likely to take him. Don't overwhelm him the first times you take him places.

Think before you go. Is this a big sale weekend at the mall? Are there likely to be huge crowds, lots of children?

It's important to begin slowly. Consider going out in public just another exercise and remember that "slow is fast." Don't be surprised if your dog behaves as if he never heard the word "sit" or "down," because in this new environment, he hasn't ever heard the words. So start at the beginning with each exercise in each new place. Your dog will catch up quickly because he's learned how to learn. But be patient. Use food and lots of praise.

Begin by practicing all the obedience exercises in your back yard. Then move into your front yard where there might be more distractions. You want to use patience and praise to keep your dog's attention on you. Follow through on each command. If you tell your dog to sit, make sure he sits. Use food treats just as you did when teaching the exercise the first time.

When your dog is obeying you promptly and consistently, go to a quiet park or schoolyard. Work several sessions, running through all the obedience commands. Remember, even if he doesn't perform an exercise as precisely as he does at home, give praise and a treat when he does it correctly. With practice he will become just as solid out in public. Don't expect perfection the first time out. It puts too much pressure on you and your dog. Strive for excellence, not perfection.

Next, go to a shopping center and work your dog in the parking lot. Be very conscious of the temperature of the pavement. Never work on blacktop when it's hot. Dogs are very sensitive to heat.

When your dog is doing his basic obedience exercises with confidence in these settings, stand with him near the entrance to a busy store. Make him sit or lie down while people pass by. If people want to pet your dog, you have the right to say yes or no. If your dog is very shy or very friendly, you should say no until you have done this exercise several times. You want this to be a positive experience and you want to maintain control. Don't let strangers crowd around your dog. Tell them he's in training as a service dog and he can't be petted. When you feel you have good control, you can allow one person to approach your dog. Your dog should not back away from or jump up to greet the person. He should remain in a sit or down stay. This may take weeks, even months, to accomplish.

If you have a shy dog, it's critical that you don't overwhelm him. You must build up his confidence very slowly and carefully to help him overcome his fear. This may take months of careful work. You may spend weeks just getting out of your car in the parking lot, then getting right back in and going home. You cannot push the shy dog. If he doesn't seem to be getting secure out in public, stop forcing him. If you push him, the stress will be too much and he may react aggressively.

If you have an aggressive dog, don't even consider taking him out in public. Even with a lot of work you can never trust a dog that has shown aggression.

If a service dog bites someone or reacts aggressively to people or dogs, it will reflect badly on service dogs everywhere. There are many people who do not want dogs around, who are just looking for an excuse to get them banned. Taking a service dog out in public is a privilege and carries with it great responsibility. Please take this responsibility seriously. If you don't trust your dog out in public, don't take him. You can still teach your shy or aggressive dog to perform many wonderful, helpful skills for you right in the comfort of your own home.

TEAMWORK

You are the only one who can decide how little or how much you want and need your dog to do for you. It takes a lot of work to teach the service exercises to your dog. You must be motivated to do it or you won't follow through. You have already accomplished a great deal just in teaching your dog basic obedience skills. Be proud of this. Keep working with your dog. Keep having fun.

If you do decide that you'd like to try to train your dog as a service dog, we will help you all we can in the book and video, TEAMWORK II. There, we go into detail on taking your dog out in public—to restaurants, work, and school. And we will teach you how to teach your dog specific skills that will help you every day.

Teamwork is really what it's all about. You and your dog are already a better team than when you started your training. Congratulations, and keep up the good work!

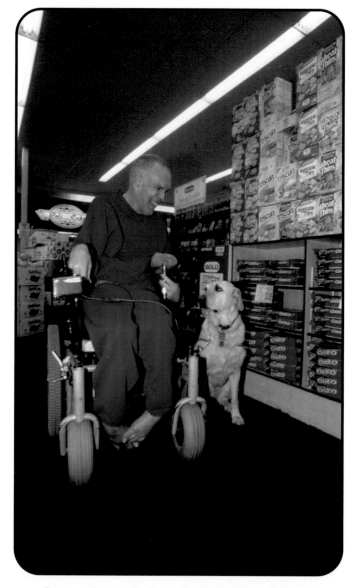

Once you have trained your dog in the basic obedience
commands, you must decide if it would be helpful and fun to train
him to the level of service dog. A service dog can accompany you
to work or school or to the store. Stewart Nordensson (cerebral
palsy) co-author of this book enjoyed taking Laura (yellow lab)
with him to the grocery store where they were well received
because she was so highly trained.